Caregiver Log

for

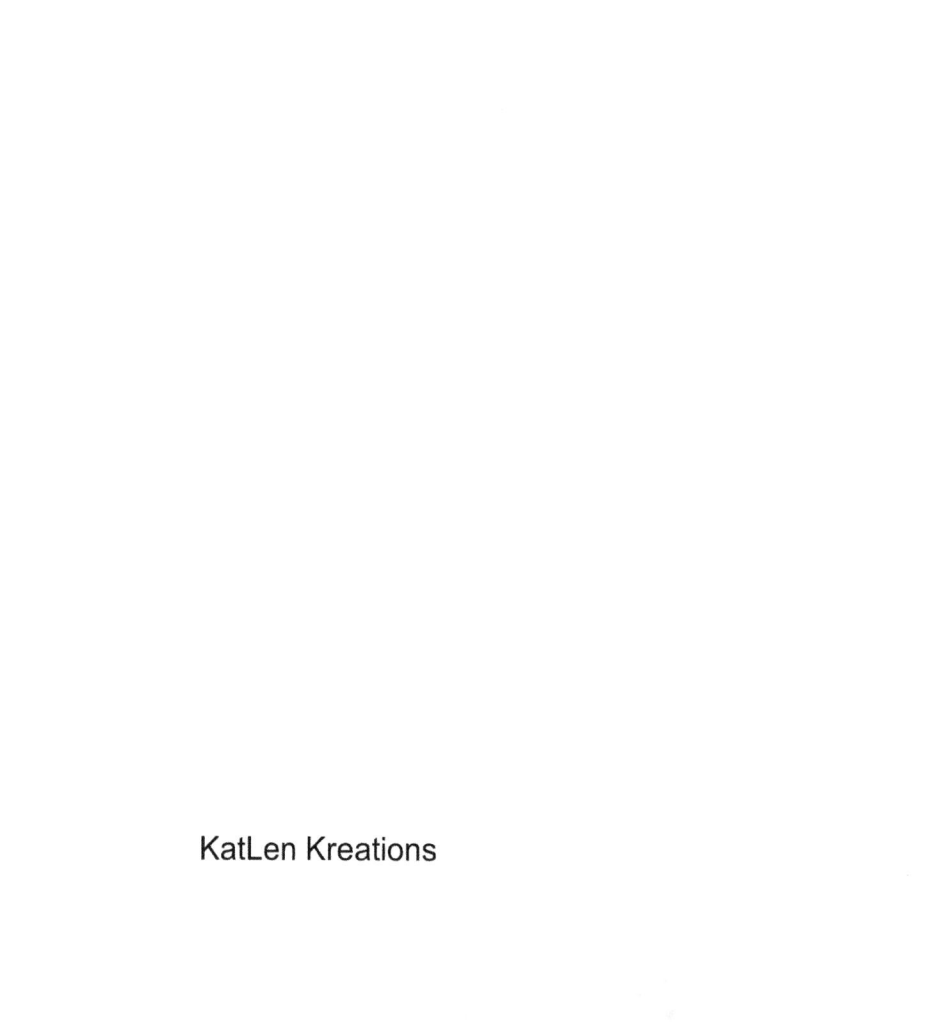

KatLen Kreations

Information Page

Name:

Contact Name and Number:

Birthday:

Health Concerns/Allergies:

Height:

Weight:

Medication	Treating	Breakfast	Lunch	Dinner	Bedtime	Other

General Notes/Additional Information

Date:

Caregivers:

Wake/Sleep

1	2	3	4	5	6	7	8	9	10	11	12	1	2	3	4	5	6	7	8	9	10	11	12

Toilet

Time:						
BM?						
Change?						

Meals: Water: ◊◊◊◊◊◊◊   Shower/Wash

Breakfast	AM snack	Lunch	PM snack	Dinner	Bedtime snack

Meds: ☐   ☐   ☐   ☐   ☐   ☐

Vitals:

Time	Blood pressure	Pulse	oxygen	Blood sugar		
	/					
	/					
	/					

Appointments or outings today: Future appointments or outings:

Visitors: Concerns/Pain Levels/Emotions:

Date: Caregivers:

Wake/Sleep

1	2	3	4	5	6	7	8	9	10	11	12	1	2	3	4	5	6	7	8	9	10	11	12

Toilet

Time:							
BM?							
Change?							

Meals: Water: ⬡⬡⬡⬡⬡⬡⬡   Shower/Wash

Breakfast	AM snack	Lunch	PM snack	Dinner	Bedtime snack

Meds: ☐   ☐   ☐   ☐   ☐   ☐

Vitals:

Time	Blood pressure	Pulse	oxygen	Blood sugar		
	/					
	/					
	/					

Appointments or outings today: Future appointments or outings:

Visitors: Concerns/Pain Levels/Emotions:

Date: _____   Caregivers: _____

Wake/Sleep

1	2	3	4	5	6	7	8	9	10	11	12	1	2	3	4	5	6	7	8	9	10	11	12

Toilet	Time:						
	BM?						
	Change?						

Meals: Water: ⬡⬡⬡⬡⬡⬡⬡   Shower/Wash

Breakfast	AM snack	Lunch	PM snack	Dinner	Bedtime snack

Meds: ☐   ☐   ☐   ☐   ☐   ☐

Vitals:

Time	Blood pressure	Pulse	oxygen	Blood sugar		
	/					
	/					
	/					

Appointments or outings today: Future appointments or outings:

Visitors: Concerns/Pain Levels/Emotions:

Date: Caregivers:

Wake/Sleep

1	2	3	4	5	6	7	8	9	10	11	12	1	2	3	4	5	6	7	8	9	10	11	12

Toilet	Time:						
	BM?						
	Change?						

Meals: Water: ⬡⬡⬡⬡⬡⬡⬡   Shower/Wash

Breakfast	AM snack	Lunch	PM snack	Dinner	Bedtime snack

Meds: ☐   ☐   ☐   ☐   ☐   ☐

Vitals:

Time	Blood pressure	Pulse	oxygen	Blood sugar		
	/					
	/					
	/					

Appointments or outings today: Future appointments or outings:

Visitors: Concerns/Pain Levels/Emotions:

Date: Caregivers:

Wake/Sleep

1	2	3	4	5	6	7	8	9	10	11	12	1	2	3	4	5	6	7	8	9	10	11	12

Toilet	Time:						
	BM?						
	Change?						

Meals: Water: ◇◇◇◇◇◇◇◇   Shower/Wash

Breakfast	AM snack	Lunch	PM snack	Dinner	Bedtime snack

Meds: ☐   ☐   ☐   ☐   ☐   ☐

Vitals:

Time	Blood pressure	Pulse	oxygen	Blood sugar		
	/					
	/					
	/					

Appointments or outings today: Future appointments or outings:

Visitors: Concerns/Pain Levels/Emotions:

Date: Caregivers:

Wake/Sleep

1	2	3	4	5	6	7	8	9	10	11	12	1	2	3	4	5	6	7	8	9	10	11	12

Toilet

Time:							
BM?							
Change?							

Meals: Water: ⬯⬯⬯⬯⬯⬯⬯   Shower/Wash

Breakfast	AM snack	Lunch	PM snack	Dinner	Bedtime snack

Meds: ☐   ☐   ☐   ☐   ☐   ☐

Vitals:

Time	Blood pressure	Pulse	oxygen	Blood sugar		
	/					
	/					
	/					

Appointments or outings today: Future appointments or outings:

Visitors: Concerns/Pain Levels/Emotions:

Date: Caregivers:

Wake/Sleep

1	2	3	4	5	6	7	8	9	10	11	12	1	2	3	4	5	6	7	8	9	10	11	12

Toilet	Time:						
	BM?						
	Change?						

Meals: Water: ◊◊◊◊◊◊◊◊ Shower/Wash

Breakfast	AM snack	Lunch	PM snack	Dinner	Bedtime snack

Meds: ☐   ☐   ☐   ☐   ☐   ☐

Vitals:

Time	Blood pressure	Pulse	oxygen	Blood sugar		
	/					
	/					
	/					

Appointments or outings today: Future appointments or outings:

Visitors: Concerns/Pain Levels/Emotions:

General Notes/Additional Information

Date: Caregivers:

Wake/Sleep

1	2	3	4	5	6	7	8	9	10	11	12	1	2	3	4	5	6	7	8	9	10	11	12

Toilet	Time:						
	BM?						
	Change?						

Meals: **Water:** ◇◇◇◇◇◇◇◇   **Shower/Wash**

Breakfast	AM snack	Lunch	PM snack	Dinner	Bedtime snack

Meds: ☐   ☐   ☐   ☐   ☐   ☐

Vitals:

Time	Blood pressure	Pulse	oxygen	Blood sugar		
	/					
	/					
	/					

Appointments or outings today: Future appointments or outings:

Visitors: Concerns/Pain Levels/Emotions:

Date: Caregivers:

Wake/Sleep

1	2	3	4	5	6	7	8	9	10	11	12	1	2	3	4	5	6	7	8	9	10	11	12

Toilet	Time:							
	BM?							
	Change?							

Meals: Water: ◊◊◊◊◊◊◊◊   Shower/Wash

Breakfast	AM snack	Lunch	PM snack	Dinner	Bedtime snack

Meds: ☐   ☐   ☐   ☐   ☐   ☐

Vitals:

Time	Blood pressure	Pulse	oxygen	Blood sugar		
	/					
	/					
	/					

Appointments or outings today: Future appointments or outings:

Visitors: Concerns/Pain Levels/Emotions:

Date: Caregivers:

Wake/Sleep

1	2	3	4	5	6	7	8	9	10	11	12	1	2	3	4	5	6	7	8	9	10	11	12

Toilet							
	Time:						
	BM?						
	Change?						

Meals: Water: ◇◇◇◇◇◇◇   Shower/Wash

Breakfast	AM snack	Lunch	PM snack	Dinner	Bedtime snack

Meds: ☐   ☐   ☐   ☐   ☐   ☐

Vitals:

Time	Blood pressure	Pulse	oxygen	Blood sugar		
	/					
	/					
	/					

Appointments or outings today: Future appointments or outings:

Visitors: Concerns/Pain Levels/Emotions:

Date: Caregivers:

Wake/Sleep

1	2	3	4	5	6	7	8	9	10	11	12	1	2	3	4	5	6	7	8	9	10	11	12

Toilet

Time:							
BM?							
Change?							

Meals: Water: ◊◊◊◊◊◊◊   Shower/Wash

Breakfast	AM snack	Lunch	PM snack	Dinner	Bedtime snack

Meds: ☐   ☐   ☐   ☐   ☐   ☐

Vitals:

Time	Blood pressure	Pulse	oxygen	Blood sugar		
	/					
	/					
	/					

Appointments or outings today: Future appointments or outings:

Visitors: Concerns/Pain Levels/Emotions:

Date: Caregivers:

Wake/Sleep

1	2	3	4	5	6	7	8	9	10	11	12	1	2	3	4	5	6	7	8	9	10	11	12

Toilet

Time:						
BM?						
Change?						

Meals: Water: ⬡⬡⬡⬡⬡⬡⬡   Shower/Wash

Breakfast	AM snack	Lunch	PM snack	Dinner	Bedtime snack

Meds: ☐   ☐   ☐   ☐   ☐   ☐

Vitals:

Time	Blood pressure	Pulse	oxygen	Blood sugar		
	/					
	/					
	/					

Appointments or outings today: Future appointments or outings:

Visitors: Concerns/Pain Levels/Emotions:

Date: Caregivers:

Wake/Sleep

1	2	3	4	5	6	7	8	9	10	11	12	1	2	3	4	5	6	7	8	9	10	11	12

Toilet	Time:							
	BM?							
	Change?							

Meals: Water: ⬡⬡⬡⬡⬡⬡⬡⬡   Shower/Wash

Breakfast	AM snack	Lunch	PM snack	Dinner	Bedtime snack

Meds: ☐   ☐   ☐   ☐   ☐   ☐

Vitals:

Time	Blood pressure	Pulse	oxygen	Blood sugar		
	/					
	/					
	/					

Appointments or outings today: Future appointments or outings:

Visitors: Concerns/Pain Levels/Emotions:

Date: Caregivers:

Wake/Sleep

1	2	3	4	5	6	7	8	9	10	11	12	1	2	3	4	5	6	7	8	9	10	11	12

Toilet	Time:						
	BM?						
	Change?						

Meals: Water: ◊◊◊◊◊◊◊   Shower/Wash

Breakfast	AM snack	Lunch	PM snack	Dinner	Bedtime snack

Meds: ☐   ☐   ☐   ☐   ☐   ☐

Vitals:

Time	Blood pressure	Pulse	oxygen	Blood sugar		
	/					
	/					
	/					

Appointments or outings today: Future appointments or outings:

Visitors: Concerns/Pain Levels/Emotions:

General Notes/Additional Information

Date: Caregivers:

Wake/Sleep

1	2	3	4	5	6	7	8	9	10	11	12	1	2	3	4	5	6	7	8	9	10	11	12

Toilet

Time:						
BM?						
Change?						

Meals: Water: ◇◇◇◇◇◇◇◇   Shower/Wash

Breakfast	AM snack	Lunch	PM snack	Dinner	Bedtime snack

Meds: ☐   ☐   ☐   ☐   ☐   ☐

Vitals:

Time	Blood pressure	Pulse	oxygen	Blood sugar		
	/					
	/					
	/					

Appointments or outings today: Future appointments or outings:

Visitors: Concerns/Pain Levels/Emotions:

Date: Caregivers:

Wake/Sleep

1	2	3	4	5	6	7	8	9	10	11	12	1	2	3	4	5	6	7	8	9	10	11	12

Toilet

Time:						
BM?						
Change?						

Meals: Water: ⬡⬡⬡⬡⬡⬡⬡   Shower/Wash

Breakfast	AM snack	Lunch	PM snack	Dinner	Bedtime snack

Meds: ☐   ☐   ☐   ☐   ☐   ☐

Vitals:

Time	Blood pressure	Pulse	oxygen	Blood sugar		
	/					
	/					
	/					

Appointments or outings today: Future appointments or outings:

Visitors: Concerns/Pain Levels/Emotions:

Date: Caregivers:

Wake/Sleep

1	2	3	4	5	6	7	8	9	10	11	12	1	2	3	4	5	6	7	8	9	10	11	12

Toilet	Time:						
	BM?						
	Change?						

Meals: Water: ◊◊◊◊◊◊◊◊   Shower/Wash

Breakfast	AM snack	Lunch	PM snack	Dinner	Bedtime snack

Meds: ☐   ☐   ☐   ☐   ☐   ☐

Vitals:

Time	Blood pressure	Pulse	oxygen	Blood sugar		
	/					
	/					
	/					

Appointments or outings today: Future appointments or outings:

Visitors: Concerns/Pain Levels/Emotions:

Date: Caregivers:

Wake/Sleep

1	2	3	4	5	6	7	8	9	10	11	12	1	2	3	4	5	6	7	8	9	10	11	12

Toilet

Time:						
BM?						
Change?						

Meals: Water: ◊◊◊◊◊◊◊   Shower/Wash

Breakfast	AM snack	Lunch	PM snack	Dinner	Bedtime snack

Meds: ☐   ☐   ☐   ☐   ☐   ☐

Vitals:

Time	Blood pressure	Pulse	oxygen	Blood sugar		
	/					
	/					
	/					

Appointments or outings today: Future appointments or outings:

Visitors: Concerns/Pain Levels/Emotions:

Date: **Caregivers:**

Wake/Sleep

1	2	3	4	5	6	7	8	9	10	11	12	1	2	3	4	5	6	7	8	9	10	11	12

Toilet

Time:						
BM?						
Change?						

Meals: **Water:** ◊◊◊◊◊◊◊◊   **Shower/Wash**

Breakfast	AM snack	Lunch	PM snack	Dinner	Bedtime snack

Meds: ☐   ☐   ☐   ☐   ☐   ☐

Vitals:

Time	Blood pressure	Pulse	oxygen	Blood sugar		
	/					
	/					
	/					

Appointments or outings today: **Future appointments or outings:**

Visitors: **Concerns/Pain Levels/Emotions:**

Date: Caregivers:

Wake/Sleep

1	2	3	4	5	6	7	8	9	10	11	12	1	2	3	4	5	6	7	8	9	10	11	12

Toilet

Time:						
BM?						
Change?						

Meals: Water: ◊◊◊◊◊◊◊   Shower/Wash

Breakfast	AM snack	Lunch	PM snack	Dinner	Bedtime snack

Meds: ☐   ☐   ☐   ☐   ☐   ☐

Vitals:

Time	Blood pressure	Pulse	oxygen	Blood sugar		
	/					
	/					
	/					

Appointments or outings today: Future appointments or outings:

Visitors: Concerns/Pain Levels/Emotions:

Date: Caregivers:

Wake/Sleep

1	2	3	4	5	6	7	8	9	10	11	12	1	2	3	4	5	6	7	8	9	10	11	12

Toilet	Time:						
	BM?						
	Change?						

Meals: Water: ◊◊◊◊◊◊◊◊   Shower/Wash

Breakfast	AM snack	Lunch	PM snack	Dinner	Bedtime snack

Meds: ☐   ☐   ☐   ☐   ☐   ☐

Vitals:

Time	Blood pressure	Pulse	oxygen	Blood sugar		
	/					
	/					
	/					

Appointments or outings today: Future appointments or outings:

Visitors: Concerns/Pain Levels/Emotions:

General Notes/Additional Information

Date: Caregivers:

Wake/Sleep

1	2	3	4	5	6	7	8	9	10	11	12	1	2	3	4	5	6	7	8	9	10	11	12

Toilet	Time:								
	BM?								
	Change?								

Meals: Water: ◊◊◊◊◊◊◊   Shower/Wash

Breakfast	AM snack	Lunch	PM snack	Dinner	Bedtime snack

Meds: ☐   ☐   ☐   ☐   ☐   ☐

Vitals:

Time	Blood pressure	Pulse	oxygen	Blood sugar		
	/					
	/					
	/					

Appointments or outings today: Future appointments or outings:

Visitors: Concerns/Pain Levels/Emotions:

Date: Caregivers:

Wake/Sleep

1	2	3	4	5	6	7	8	9	10	11	12	1	2	3	4	5	6	7	8	9	10	11	12

Toilet	Time:						
	BM?						
	Change?						

Meals: Water: ⬦⬦⬦⬦⬦⬦⬦   Shower/Wash

Breakfast	AM snack	Lunch	PM snack	Dinner	Bedtime snack

Meds: ☐   ☐   ☐   ☐   ☐   ☐

Vitals:

Time	Blood pressure	Pulse	oxygen	Blood sugar		
	/					
	/					
	/					

Appointments or outings today: Future appointments or outings:

Visitors: Concerns/Pain Levels/Emotions:

Date: Caregivers:

Wake/Sleep

1	2	3	4	5	6	7	8	9	10	11	12	1	2	3	4	5	6	7	8	9	10	11	12

Toilet	Time:						
	BM?						
	Change?						

Meals: Water: ◊◊◊◊◊◊◊   Shower/Wash

Breakfast	AM snack	Lunch	PM snack	Dinner	Bedtime snack

Meds: ☐   ☐   ☐   ☐   ☐   ☐

Vitals:

Time	Blood pressure	Pulse	oxygen	Blood sugar		
	/					
	/					
	/					

Appointments or outings today: Future appointments or outings:

Visitors: Concerns/Pain Levels/Emotions:

Date: Caregivers:

Wake/Sleep

1	2	3	4	5	6	7	8	9	10	11	12	1	2	3	4	5	6	7	8	9	10	11	12

Toilet	Time:						
	BM?						
	Change?						

Meals: Water: ⬡⬡⬡⬡⬡⬡⬡   Shower/Wash

Breakfast	AM snack	Lunch	PM snack	Dinner	Bedtime snack

Meds: ☐   ☐   ☐   ☐   ☐   ☐

Vitals:

Time	Blood pressure	Pulse	oxygen	Blood sugar		
	/					
	/					
	/					

Appointments or outings today: Future appointments or outings:

Visitors: Concerns/Pain Levels/Emotions:

Date: Caregivers:

Wake/Sleep

1	2	3	4	5	6	7	8	9	10	11	12	1	2	3	4	5	6	7	8	9	10	11	12

Toilet	Time:						
	BM?						
	Change?						

Meals: Water: ◊◊◊◊◊◊◊◊   Shower/Wash

Breakfast	AM snack	Lunch	PM snack	Dinner	Bedtime snack

Meds: ☐   ☐   ☐   ☐   ☐   ☐

Vitals:

Time	Blood pressure	Pulse	oxygen	Blood sugar		
	/					
	/					
	/					

Appointments or outings today: Future appointments or outings:

Visitors: Concerns/Pain Levels/Emotions:

Date: Caregivers:

Wake/Sleep

1	2	3	4	5	6	7	8	9	10	11	12	1	2	3	4	5	6	7	8	9	10	11	12

Toilet	Time:						
	BM?						
	Change?						

Meals: Water: ⬠⬠⬠⬠⬠⬠⬠⬠   Shower/Wash

Breakfast	AM snack	Lunch	PM snack	Dinner	Bedtime snack

Meds: ☐   ☐   ☐   ☐   ☐   ☐

Vitals:

Time	Blood pressure	Pulse	oxygen	Blood sugar		
	/					
	/					
	/					

Appointments or outings today: Future appointments or outings:

Visitors: Concerns/Pain Levels/Emotions:

Date: Caregivers:

Wake/Sleep

1	2	3	4	5	6	7	8	9	10	11	12	1	2	3	4	5	6	7	8	9	10	11	12

Toilet	Time:						
	BM?						
	Change?						

Meals: Water: ◊◊◊◊◊◊◊   Shower/Wash

Breakfast	AM snack	Lunch	PM snack	Dinner	Bedtime snack

Meds: ☐   ☐   ☐   ☐   ☐   ☐

Vitals:

Time	Blood pressure	Pulse	oxygen	Blood sugar		
	/					
	/					
	/					

Appointments or outings today: Future appointments or outings:

Visitors: Concerns/Pain Levels/Emotions:

General Notes/Additional Information

Date: Caregivers:

Wake/Sleep

1	2	3	4	5	6	7	8	9	10	11	12	1	2	3	4	5	6	7	8	9	10	11	12

Toilet	Time:						
	BM?						
	Change?						

Meals: Water: ◊◊◊◊◊◊◊   Shower/Wash

Breakfast	AM snack	Lunch	PM snack	Dinner	Bedtime snack

Meds: ☐   ☐   ☐   ☐   ☐   ☐

Vitals:

Time	Blood pressure	Pulse	oxygen	Blood sugar		
	/					
	/					
	/					

Appointments or outings today: Future appointments or outings:

Visitors: Concerns/Pain Levels/Emotions:

Date: Caregivers:

Wake/Sleep

1	2	3	4	5	6	7	8	9	10	11	12	1	2	3	4	5	6	7	8	9	10	11	12

Toilet	Time:						
	BM?						
	Change?						

Meals: Water: ⬭⬭⬭⬭⬭⬭⬭   Shower/Wash

Breakfast	AM snack	Lunch	PM snack	Dinner	Bedtime snack

Meds: ☐   ☐   ☐   ☐   ☐   ☐

Vitals:

Time	Blood pressure	Pulse	oxygen	Blood sugar		
	/					
	/					
	/					

Appointments or outings today: Future appointments or outings:

Visitors: Concerns/Pain Levels/Emotions:

Date: Caregivers:

Wake/Sleep

1	2	3	4	5	6	7	8	9	10	11	12	1	2	3	4	5	6	7	8	9	10	11	12

Toilet

Time:						
BM?						
Change?						

Meals: Water: ⬠⬠⬠⬠⬠⬠⬠   Shower/Wash

Breakfast	AM snack	Lunch	PM snack	Dinner	Bedtime snack

Meds: ☐   ☐   ☐   ☐   ☐   ☐

Vitals:

Time	Blood pressure	Pulse	oxygen	Blood sugar		
	/					
	/					
	/					

Appointments or outings today: Future appointments or outings:

Visitors: Concerns/Pain Levels/Emotions:

Date: Caregivers:

Wake/Sleep

1	2	3	4	5	6	7	8	9	10	11	12	1	2	3	4	5	6	7	8	9	10	11	12

Toilet

Time:						
BM?						
Change?						

Meals: Water: ⬭⬭⬭⬭⬭⬭⬭   Shower/Wash

Breakfast	AM snack	Lunch	PM snack	Dinner	Bedtime snack

Meds: ☐   ☐   ☐   ☐   ☐   ☐

Vitals:

Time	Blood pressure	Pulse	oxygen	Blood sugar		
	/					
	/					
	/					

Appointments or outings today: Future appointments or outings:

Visitors: Concerns/Pain Levels/Emotions:

Date: Caregivers:

Wake/Sleep

1	2	3	4	5	6	7	8	9	10	11	12	1	2	3	4	5	6	7	8	9	10	11	12

Toilet	Time:							
	BM?							
	Change?							

Meals: Water: ◊◊◊◊◊◊◊◊   Shower/Wash

Breakfast	AM snack	Lunch	PM snack	Dinner	Bedtime snack

Meds: ☐   ☐   ☐   ☐   ☐   ☐

Vitals:

Time	Blood pressure	Pulse	oxygen	Blood sugar		
	/					
	/					
	/					

Appointments or outings today: Future appointments or outings:

Visitors: Concerns/Pain Levels/Emotions:

Date: Caregivers:

Wake/Sleep

1	2	3	4	5	6	7	8	9	10	11	12	1	2	3	4	5	6	7	8	9	10	11	12

Toilet

Time:						
BM?						
Change?						

Meals: Water: ⬭⬭⬭⬭⬭⬭⬭⬭   Shower/Wash

Breakfast	AM snack	Lunch	PM snack	Dinner	Bedtime snack

Meds: ☐   ☐   ☐   ☐   ☐   ☐

Vitals:

Time	Blood pressure	Pulse	oxygen	Blood sugar		
	/					
	/					
	/					

Appointments or outings today: Future appointments or outings:

Visitors: Concerns/Pain Levels/Emotions:

Date: **Caregivers:**

Wake/Sleep

1	2	3	4	5	6	7	8	9	10	11	12	1	2	3	4	5	6	7	8	9	10	11	12

Toilet	Time:						
	BM?						
	Change?						

Meals: Water: ⬡⬡⬡⬡⬡⬡⬡   Shower/Wash

Breakfast	AM snack	Lunch	PM snack	Dinner	Bedtime snack

Meds: ☐   ☐   ☐   ☐   ☐   ☐

Vitals:

Time	Blood pressure	Pulse	oxygen	Blood sugar		
	/					
	/					
	/					

Appointments or outings today: Future appointments or outings:

Visitors: Concerns/Pain Levels/Emotions:

General Notes/Additional Information

Date: Caregivers:

Wake/Sleep

1	2	3	4	5	6	7	8	9	10	11	12	1	2	3	4	5	6	7	8	9	10	11	12

Toilet

Time:							
BM?							
Change?							

Meals: Water: ◊◊◊◊◊◊◊   Shower/Wash

Breakfast	AM snack	Lunch	PM snack	Dinner	Bedtime snack

Meds: ☐   ☐   ☐   ☐   ☐   ☐

Vitals:

Time	Blood pressure	Pulse	oxygen	Blood sugar		
	/					
	/					
	/					

Appointments or outings today: Future appointments or outings:

Visitors: Concerns/Pain Levels/Emotions:

Date: Caregivers:

Wake/Sleep

1	2	3	4	5	6	7	8	9	10	11	12	1	2	3	4	5	6	7	8	9	10	11	12

Toilet

Time:							
BM?							
Change?							

Meals: Water: ⬡⬡⬡⬡⬡⬡⬡   Shower/Wash

Breakfast	AM snack	Lunch	PM snack	Dinner	Bedtime snack

Meds: ☐   ☐   ☐   ☐   ☐   ☐

Vitals:

Time	Blood pressure	Pulse	oxygen	Blood sugar		
	/					
	/					
	/					

Appointments or outings today: Future appointments or outings:

Visitors: Concerns/Pain Levels/Emotions:

Date: Caregivers:

Wake/Sleep

1	2	3	4	5	6	7	8	9	10	11	12	1	2	3	4	5	6	7	8	9	10	11	12

Toilet
Time:						
BM?						
Change?						

Meals: Water: ◊◊◊◊◊◊◊◊   Shower/Wash

Breakfast	AM snack	Lunch	PM snack	Dinner	Bedtime snack

Meds: ☐   ☐   ☐   ☐   ☐   ☐

Vitals:

Time	Blood pressure	Pulse	oxygen	Blood sugar		
	/					
	/					
	/					

Appointments or outings today: Future appointments or outings:

Visitors: Concerns/Pain Levels/Emotions:

Date: Caregivers:

Wake/Sleep

1	2	3	4	5	6	7	8	9	10	11	12	1	2	3	4	5	6	7	8	9	10	11	12

Toilet

Time:							
BM?							
Change?							

Meals: Water: ⬡⬡⬡⬡⬡⬡⬡   Shower/Wash

Breakfast	AM snack	Lunch	PM snack	Dinner	Bedtime snack

Meds: ☐   ☐   ☐   ☐   ☐   ☐

Vitals:

Time	Blood pressure	Pulse	oxygen	Blood sugar		
	/					
	/					
	/					

Appointments or outings today: Future appointments or outings:

Visitors: Concerns/Pain Levels/Emotions:

Date: Caregivers:

Wake/Sleep

1	2	3	4	5	6	7	8	9	10	11	12	1	2	3	4	5	6	7	8	9	10	11	12

Toilet	Time:							
	BM?							
	Change?							

Meals: Water: ◊◊◊◊◊◊◊◊   Shower/Wash

Breakfast	AM snack	Lunch	PM snack	Dinner	Bedtime snack

Meds: ☐   ☐   ☐   ☐   ☐   ☐

Vitals:

Time	Blood pressure	Pulse	oxygen	Blood sugar		
	/					
	/					
	/					

Appointments or outings today: Future appointments or outings:

Visitors: Concerns/Pain Levels/Emotions:

Date: Caregivers:

Wake/Sleep

1	2	3	4	5	6	7	8	9	10	11	12	1	2	3	4	5	6	7	8	9	10	11	12

Toilet

Time:						
BM?						
Change?						

Meals: Water: ⬦⬦⬦⬦⬦⬦⬦   Shower/Wash

Breakfast	AM snack	Lunch	PM snack	Dinner	Bedtime snack

Meds: ☐   ☐   ☐   ☐   ☐   ☐

Vitals:

Time	Blood pressure	Pulse	oxygen	Blood sugar		
	/					
	/					
	/					

Appointments or outings today: Future appointments or outings:

Visitors: Concerns/Pain Levels/Emotions:

Date: **Caregivers:**

Wake/Sleep

1	2	3	4	5	6	7	8	9	10	11	12	1	2	3	4	5	6	7	8	9	10	11	12

Toilet	Time:						
	BM?						
	Change?						

Meals: Water: ⬭⬭⬭⬭⬭⬭⬭   Shower/Wash

Breakfast	AM snack	Lunch	PM snack	Dinner	Bedtime snack

Meds: ☐   ☐   ☐   ☐   ☐   ☐

Vitals:

Time	Blood pressure	Pulse	oxygen	Blood sugar		
	/					
	/					
	/					

Appointments or outings today: Future appointments or outings:

Visitors: Concerns/Pain Levels/Emotions:

General Notes/Additional Information

Date: Caregivers:

Wake/Sleep

1	2	3	4	5	6	7	8	9	10	11	12	1	2	3	4	5	6	7	8	9	10	11	12

Toilet	Time:						
	BM?						
	Change?						

Meals: Water: ◊◊◊◊◊◊◊◊   Shower/Wash

Breakfast	AM snack	Lunch	PM snack	Dinner	Bedtime snack

Meds: ☐   ☐   ☐   ☐   ☐   ☐

Vitals:

Time	Blood pressure	Pulse	oxygen	Blood sugar		
	/					
	/					
	/					

Appointments or outings today: Future appointments or outings:

Visitors: Concerns/Pain Levels/Emotions:

Date: Caregivers:

Wake/Sleep

1	2	3	4	5	6	7	8	9	10	11	12	1	2	3	4	5	6	7	8	9	10	11	12

Toilet	Time:						
	BM?						
	Change?						

Meals: Water: ⬭⬭⬭⬭⬭⬭⬭⬭   Shower/Wash

Breakfast	AM snack	Lunch	PM snack	Dinner	Bedtime snack

Meds: ☐   ☐   ☐   ☐   ☐   ☐

Vitals:

Time	Blood pressure	Pulse	oxygen	Blood sugar		
	/					
	/					
	/					

Appointments or outings today: Future appointments or outings:

Visitors: Concerns/Pain Levels/Emotions:

Date: Caregivers:

Wake/Sleep

1	2	3	4	5	6	7	8	9	10	11	12	1	2	3	4	5	6	7	8	9	10	11	12

Toilet	Time:						
	BM?						
	Change?						

Meals: Water: ⬡⬡⬡⬡⬡⬡⬡   Shower/Wash

Breakfast	AM snack	Lunch	PM snack	Dinner	Bedtime snack

Meds: ☐   ☐   ☐   ☐   ☐   ☐

Vitals:

Time	Blood pressure	Pulse	oxygen	Blood sugar		
	/					
	/					
	/					

Appointments or outings today: Future appointments or outings:

Visitors: Concerns/Pain Levels/Emotions:

Date: Caregivers:

Wake/Sleep

1	2	3	4	5	6	7	8	9	10	11	12	1	2	3	4	5	6	7	8	9	10	11	12

Toilet	Time:						
	BM?						
	Change?						

Meals: Water: ⬡⬡⬡⬡⬡⬡⬡   Shower/Wash

Breakfast	AM snack	Lunch	PM snack	Dinner	Bedtime snack

Meds: ☐   ☐   ☐   ☐   ☐   ☐

Vitals:

Time	Blood pressure	Pulse	oxygen	Blood sugar		
	/					
	/					
	/					

Appointments or outings today: Future appointments or outings:

Visitors: Concerns/Pain Levels/Emotions:

Date: _____   Caregivers: _____

Wake/Sleep

1	2	3	4	5	6	7	8	9	10	11	12	1	2	3	4	5	6	7	8	9	10	11	12

Toilet	Time:						
	BM?						
	Change?						

Meals: Water: ⬡⬡⬡⬡⬡⬡⬡   Shower/Wash

Breakfast	AM snack	Lunch	PM snack	Dinner	Bedtime snack

Meds: ☐   ☐   ☐   ☐   ☐   ☐

Vitals:

Time	Blood pressure	Pulse	oxygen	Blood sugar		
	/					
	/					
	/					

Appointments or outings today: Future appointments or outings:

Visitors: Concerns/Pain Levels/Emotions:

Date: Caregivers:

Wake/Sleep

1	2	3	4	5	6	7	8	9	10	11	12	1	2	3	4	5	6	7	8	9	10	11	12

Toilet	Time:						
	BM?						
	Change?						

Meals: Water: ⬦⬦⬦⬦⬦⬦⬦   Shower/Wash

Breakfast	AM snack	Lunch	PM snack	Dinner	Bedtime snack

Meds: ☐   ☐   ☐   ☐   ☐   ☐

Vitals:

Time	Blood pressure	Pulse	oxygen	Blood sugar		
	/					
	/					
	/					

Appointments or outings today: Future appointments or outings:

Visitors: Concerns/Pain Levels/Emotions:

Date: Caregivers:

Wake/Sleep

1	2	3	4	5	6	7	8	9	10	11	12	1	2	3	4	5	6	7	8	9	10	11	12

Toilet	Time:						
	BM?						
	Change?						

Meals: Water: ⬭⬭⬭⬭⬭⬭⬭   Shower/Wash

Breakfast	AM snack	Lunch	PM snack	Dinner	Bedtime snack

Meds: ☐   ☐   ☐   ☐   ☐   ☐

Vitals:

Time	Blood pressure	Pulse	oxygen	Blood sugar		
	/					
	/					
	/					

Appointments or outings today: Future appointments or outings:

Visitors: Concerns/Pain Levels/Emotions:

General Notes/Additional Information

Date: Caregivers:

Wake/Sleep

1	2	3	4	5	6	7	8	9	10	11	12	1	2	3	4	5	6	7	8	9	10	11	12

Toilet	Time:						
	BM?						
	Change?						

Meals: Water: ⬡⬡⬡⬡⬡⬡⬡   Shower/Wash

Breakfast	AM snack	Lunch	PM snack	Dinner	Bedtime snack

Meds: ☐   ☐   ☐   ☐   ☐   ☐

Vitals:

Time	Blood pressure	Pulse	oxygen	Blood sugar		
	/					
	/					
	/					

Appointments or outings today: Future appointments or outings:

Visitors: Concerns/Pain Levels/Emotions:

Date: Caregivers:

Wake/Sleep

1	2	3	4	5	6	7	8	9	10	11	12	1	2	3	4	5	6	7	8	9	10	11	12

Toilet

Time:							
BM?							
Change?							

Meals: Water: ⬡⬡⬡⬡⬡⬡⬡   Shower/Wash

Breakfast	AM snack	Lunch	PM snack	Dinner	Bedtime snack

Meds: ☐   ☐   ☐   ☐   ☐   ☐

Vitals:

Time	Blood pressure	Pulse	oxygen	Blood sugar		
	/					
	/					
	/					

Appointments or outings today: Future appointments or outings:

Visitors: Concerns/Pain Levels/Emotions:

Date: Caregivers:

Wake/Sleep

1	2	3	4	5	6	7	8	9	10	11	12	1	2	3	4	5	6	7	8	9	10	11	12

Toilet	Time:							
	BM?							
	Change?							

Meals: Water: ◌◌◌◌◌◌◌◌   Shower/Wash

Breakfast	AM snack	Lunch	PM snack	Dinner	Bedtime snack

Meds: ☐   ☐   ☐   ☐   ☐   ☐

Vitals:

Time	Blood pressure	Pulse	oxygen	Blood sugar		
	/					
	/					
	/					

Appointments or outings today: Future appointments or outings:

Visitors: Concerns/Pain Levels/Emotions:

Date: Caregivers:

Wake/Sleep

1	2	3	4	5	6	7	8	9	10	11	12	1	2	3	4	5	6	7	8	9	10	11	12

Toilet	Time:						
	BM?						
	Change?						

Meals: Water: ⬡⬡⬡⬡⬡⬡⬡   Shower/Wash

Breakfast	AM snack	Lunch	PM snack	Dinner	Bedtime snack

Meds: ☐   ☐   ☐   ☐   ☐   ☐

Vitals:

Time	Blood pressure	Pulse	oxygen	Blood sugar		
	/					
	/					
	/					

Appointments or outings today: Future appointments or outings:

Visitors: Concerns/Pain Levels/Emotions:

Date: Caregivers:

Wake/Sleep

1	2	3	4	5	6	7	8	9	10	11	12	1	2	3	4	5	6	7	8	9	10	11	12

Toilet	Time:						
	BM?						
	Change?						

Meals: Water: ⬭⬭⬭⬭⬭⬭⬭   Shower/Wash

Breakfast	AM snack	Lunch	PM snack	Dinner	Bedtime snack

Meds: ☐   ☐   ☐   ☐   ☐   ☐

Vitals:

Time	Blood pressure	Pulse	oxygen	Blood sugar		
	/					
	/					
	/					

Appointments or outings today: Future appointments or outings:

Visitors: Concerns/Pain Levels/Emotions:

Date: Caregivers:

Wake/Sleep

1	2	3	4	5	6	7	8	9	10	11	12	1	2	3	4	5	6	7	8	9	10	11	12

Toilet	Time:						
	BM?						
	Change?						

Meals: Water: ⬡⬡⬡⬡⬡⬡⬡⬡   Shower/Wash

Breakfast	AM snack	Lunch	PM snack	Dinner	Bedtime snack

Meds: ☐   ☐   ☐   ☐   ☐   ☐

Vitals:

Time	Blood pressure	Pulse	oxygen	Blood sugar		
	/					
	/					
	/					

Appointments or outings today: Future appointments or outings:

Visitors: Concerns/Pain Levels/Emotions:

Date: **Caregivers:**

Wake/Sleep

1	2	3	4	5	6	7	8	9	10	11	12	1	2	3	4	5	6	7	8	9	10	11	12

Toilet							
	Time:						
	BM?						
	Change?						

Meals: Water: ◊◊◊◊◊◊◊   Shower/Wash

Breakfast	AM snack	Lunch	PM snack	Dinner	Bedtime snack

Meds: ☐   ☐   ☐   ☐   ☐   ☐

Vitals:

Time	Blood pressure	Pulse	oxygen	Blood sugar		
	/					
	/					
	/					

Appointments or outings today: Future appointments or outings:

Visitors: Concerns/Pain Levels/Emotions:

General Notes/Additional Information

Date: Caregivers:

Wake/Sleep

1	2	3	4	5	6	7	8	9	10	11	12	1	2	3	4	5	6	7	8	9	10	11	12

Toilet	Time:							
	BM?							
	Change?							

Meals: Water: ⬡⬡⬡⬡⬡⬡⬡   Shower/Wash

Breakfast	AM snack	Lunch	PM snack	Dinner	Bedtime snack

Meds: ☐   ☐   ☐   ☐   ☐   ☐

Vitals:

Time	Blood pressure	Pulse	oxygen	Blood sugar		
	/					
	/					
	/					

Appointments or outings today: Future appointments or outings:

Visitors: Concerns/Pain Levels/Emotions:

Date: Caregivers:

Wake/Sleep

1	2	3	4	5	6	7	8	9	10	11	12	1	2	3	4	5	6	7	8	9	10	11	12

Toilet

Time:						
BM?						
Change?						

Meals: Water: ⬡⬡⬡⬡⬡⬡⬡   Shower/Wash

Breakfast	AM snack	Lunch	PM snack	Dinner	Bedtime snack

Meds: ☐   ☐   ☐   ☐   ☐   ☐

Vitals:

Time	Blood pressure	Pulse	oxygen	Blood sugar		
	/					
	/					
	/					

Appointments or outings today: Future appointments or outings:

Visitors: Concerns/Pain Levels/Emotions:

Date: Caregivers:

Wake/Sleep

1	2	3	4	5	6	7	8	9	10	11	12	1	2	3	4	5	6	7	8	9	10	11	12

Toilet

Time:						
BM?						
Change?						

Meals: Water: ⬭⬭⬭⬭⬭⬭⬭⬭   Shower/Wash

Breakfast	AM snack	Lunch	PM snack	Dinner	Bedtime snack

Meds: ☐   ☐   ☐   ☐   ☐   ☐

Vitals:

Time	Blood pressure	Pulse	oxygen	Blood sugar		
	/					
	/					
	/					

Appointments or outings today: Future appointments or outings:

Visitors: Concerns/Pain Levels/Emotions:

Date: **Caregivers:**

Wake/Sleep

1	2	3	4	5	6	7	8	9	10	11	12	1	2	3	4	5	6	7	8	9	10	11	12

Toilet

Time:						
BM?						
Change?						

Meals:　　　　　　　　　　Water: ◊◊◊◊◊◊◊◊　　　　Shower/Wash

Breakfast	AM snack	Lunch	PM snack	Dinner	Bedtime snack

Meds: ☐　　　☐　　　☐　　　☐　　　☐　　　☐

Vitals:

Time	Blood pressure	Pulse	oxygen	Blood sugar		
	/					
	/					
	/					

Appointments or outings today:　　　　　　　Future appointments or outings:

Visitors:　　　　　　　　　　　　　　　　Concerns/Pain Levels/Emotions:

Date: _____   Caregivers: _____

Wake/Sleep

1	2	3	4	5	6	7	8	9	10	11	12	1	2	3	4	5	6	7	8	9	10	11	12

Toilet	Time:						
	BM?						
	Change?						

Meals: Water: ◊◊◊◊◊◊◊◊   Shower/Wash

Breakfast	AM snack	Lunch	PM snack	Dinner	Bedtime snack

Meds: ☐   ☐   ☐   ☐   ☐   ☐

Vitals:

Time	Blood pressure	Pulse	oxygen	Blood sugar		
	/					
	/					
	/					

Appointments or outings today: Future appointments or outings:

Visitors: Concerns/Pain Levels/Emotions:

Date: Caregivers:

Wake/Sleep

1	2	3	4	5	6	7	8	9	10	11	12	1	2	3	4	5	6	7	8	9	10	11	12

Toilet

Time:						
BM?						
Change?						

Meals: Water: ⬭⬭⬭⬭⬭⬭⬭   Shower/Wash

Breakfast	AM snack	Lunch	PM snack	Dinner	Bedtime snack

Meds: ☐   ☐   ☐   ☐   ☐   ☐

Vitals:

Time	Blood pressure	Pulse	oxygen	Blood sugar		
	/					
	/					
	/					

Appointments or outings today: Future appointments or outings:

Visitors: Concerns/Pain Levels/Emotions:

Date: **Caregivers:**

Wake/Sleep

1	2	3	4	5	6	7	8	9	10	11	12	1	2	3	4	5	6	7	8	9	10	11	12

Toilet	Time:						
	BM?						
	Change?						

Meals: **Water:** ⬡⬡⬡⬡⬡⬡⬡⬡   **Shower/Wash**

Breakfast	AM snack	Lunch	PM snack	Dinner	Bedtime snack

Meds: ☐   ☐   ☐   ☐   ☐   ☐

Vitals:

Time	Blood pressure	Pulse	oxygen	Blood sugar		
	/					
	/					
	/					

Appointments or outings today: **Future appointments or outings:**

Visitors: **Concerns/Pain Levels/Emotions:**

General Notes/Additional Information

Date: Caregivers:

Wake/Sleep

1	2	3	4	5	6	7	8	9	10	11	12	1	2	3	4	5	6	7	8	9	10	11	12

Toilet	Time:						
	BM?						
	Change?						

Meals: Water: ⬭⬭⬭⬭⬭⬭⬭   Shower/Wash

Breakfast	AM snack	Lunch	PM snack	Dinner	Bedtime snack

Meds: ☐   ☐   ☐   ☐   ☐   ☐

Vitals:

Time	Blood pressure	Pulse	oxygen	Blood sugar		
	/					
	/					
	/					

Appointments or outings today: Future appointments or outings:

Visitors: Concerns/Pain Levels/Emotions:

Date: Caregivers:

Wake/Sleep

1	2	3	4	5	6	7	8	9	10	11	12	1	2	3	4	5	6	7	8	9	10	11	12

Toilet	Time:							
	BM?							
	Change?							

Meals: Water: ⬡⬡⬡⬡⬡⬡⬡ Shower/Wash

Breakfast	AM snack	Lunch	PM snack	Dinner	Bedtime snack

Meds: ☐ ☐ ☐ ☐ ☐ ☐

Vitals:

Time	Blood pressure	Pulse	oxygen	Blood sugar		
	/					
	/					
	/					

Appointments or outings today: Future appointments or outings:

Visitors: Concerns/Pain Levels/Emotions:

Date: Caregivers:

Wake/Sleep

1	2	3	4	5	6	7	8	9	10	11	12	1	2	3	4	5	6	7	8	9	10	11	12

Toilet	Time:						
	BM?						
	Change?						

Meals: Water: ⬭⬭⬭⬭⬭⬭⬭   Shower/Wash

Breakfast	AM snack	Lunch	PM snack	Dinner	Bedtime snack

Meds: ☐   ☐   ☐   ☐   ☐   ☐

Vitals:

Time	Blood pressure	Pulse	oxygen	Blood sugar		
	/					
	/					
	/					

Appointments or outings today: Future appointments or outings:

Visitors: Concerns/Pain Levels/Emotions:

Date: Caregivers:

Wake/Sleep

1	2	3	4	5	6	7	8	9	10	11	12	1	2	3	4	5	6	7	8	9	10	11	12

Toilet	Time:						
	BM?						
	Change?						

Meals: Water: ⬯⬯⬯⬯⬯⬯⬯   Shower/Wash

Breakfast	AM snack	Lunch	PM snack	Dinner	Bedtime snack

Meds: ☐   ☐   ☐   ☐   ☐   ☐

Vitals:

Time	Blood pressure	Pulse	oxygen	Blood sugar		
	/					
	/					
	/					

Appointments or outings today: Future appointments or outings:

Visitors: Concerns/Pain Levels/Emotions:

Date: **Caregivers:**

Wake/Sleep

1	2	3	4	5	6	7	8	9	10	11	12	1	2	3	4	5	6	7	8	9	10	11	12

Toilet

Time:						
BM?						
Change?						

Meals: **Water:** ⬡⬡⬡⬡⬡⬡⬡   **Shower/Wash**

Breakfast	AM snack	Lunch	PM snack	Dinner	Bedtime snack

Meds: ☐   ☐   ☐   ☐   ☐   ☐

Vitals:

Time	Blood pressure	Pulse	oxygen	Blood sugar		
	/					
	/					
	/					

Appointments or outings today: **Future appointments or outings:**

Visitors: **Concerns/Pain Levels/Emotions:**

Date: **Caregivers:**

Wake/Sleep

1	2	3	4	5	6	7	8	9	10	11	12	1	2	3	4	5	6	7	8	9	10	11	12

Toilet

Time:							
BM?							
Change?							

Meals: Water: ⬦⬦⬦⬦⬦⬦⬦   Shower/Wash

Breakfast	AM snack	Lunch	PM snack	Dinner	Bedtime snack

Meds: ☐   ☐   ☐   ☐   ☐   ☐

Vitals:

Time	Blood pressure	Pulse	oxygen	Blood sugar		
	/					
	/					
	/					

Appointments or outings today: Future appointments or outings:

Visitors: Concerns/Pain Levels/Emotions:

Date: Caregivers:

Wake/Sleep

1	2	3	4	5	6	7	8	9	10	11	12	1	2	3	4	5	6	7	8	9	10	11	12

Toilet

Time:						
BM?						
Change?						

Meals: Water: ⬡⬡⬡⬡⬡⬡⬡   Shower/Wash

Breakfast	AM snack	Lunch	PM snack	Dinner	Bedtime snack

Meds: ☐   ☐   ☐   ☐   ☐   ☐

Vitals:

Time	Blood pressure	Pulse	oxygen	Blood sugar		
	/					
	/					
	/					

Appointments or outings today: Future appointments or outings:

Visitors: Concerns/Pain Levels/Emotions:

General Notes/Additional Information

Date: Caregivers:

Wake/Sleep

1	2	3	4	5	6	7	8	9	10	11	12	1	2	3	4	5	6	7	8	9	10	11	12

Toilet	Time:							
	BM?							
	Change?							

Meals: Water: ◊◊◊◊◊◊◊   Shower/Wash

Breakfast	AM snack	Lunch	PM snack	Dinner	Bedtime snack

Meds: ☐   ☐   ☐   ☐   ☐   ☐

Vitals:

Time	Blood pressure	Pulse	oxygen	Blood sugar		
	/					
	/					
	/					

Appointments or outings today: Future appointments or outings:

Visitors: Concerns/Pain Levels/Emotions:

Date: Caregivers:

Wake/Sleep

1	2	3	4	5	6	7	8	9	10	11	12	1	2	3	4	5	6	7	8	9	10	11	12

Toilet

Time:							
BM?							
Change?							

Meals: Water: ◊◊◊◊◊◊◊◊   Shower/Wash

Breakfast	AM snack	Lunch	PM snack	Dinner	Bedtime snack

Meds: ☐   ☐   ☐   ☐   ☐   ☐

Vitals:

Time	Blood pressure	Pulse	oxygen	Blood sugar		
	/					
	/					
	/					

Appointments or outings today: Future appointments or outings:

Visitors: Concerns/Pain Levels/Emotions:

Date: Caregivers:

Wake/Sleep

1	2	3	4	5	6	7	8	9	10	11	12	1	2	3	4	5	6	7	8	9	10	11	12

Toilet	Time:						
	BM?						
	Change?						

Meals: Water: ⬡⬡⬡⬡⬡⬡⬡⬡   Shower/Wash

Breakfast	AM snack	Lunch	PM snack	Dinner	Bedtime snack

Meds: ☐   ☐   ☐   ☐   ☐   ☐

Vitals:

Time	Blood pressure	Pulse	oxygen	Blood sugar		
	/					
	/					
	/					

Appointments or outings today: Future appointments or outings:

Visitors: Concerns/Pain Levels/Emotions:

Date: Caregivers:

Wake/Sleep

1	2	3	4	5	6	7	8	9	10	11	12	1	2	3	4	5	6	7	8	9	10	11	12

Toilet

Time:						
BM?						
Change?						

Meals: Water: ⬭⬭⬭⬭⬭⬭⬭   Shower/Wash

Breakfast	AM snack	Lunch	PM snack	Dinner	Bedtime snack

Meds: ☐   ☐   ☐   ☐   ☐   ☐

Vitals:

Time	Blood pressure	Pulse	oxygen	Blood sugar		
	/					
	/					
	/					

Appointments or outings today: Future appointments or outings:

Visitors: Concerns/Pain Levels/Emotions:

Date: Caregivers:

Wake/Sleep

1	2	3	4	5	6	7	8	9	10	11	12	1	2	3	4	5	6	7	8	9	10	11	12

Toilet

Time:						
BM?						
Change?						

Meals: Water: ◊◊◊◊◊◊◊   Shower/Wash

Breakfast	AM snack	Lunch	PM snack	Dinner	Bedtime snack

Meds: ☐   ☐   ☐   ☐   ☐   ☐

Vitals:

Time	Blood pressure	Pulse	oxygen	Blood sugar		
	/					
	/					
	/					

Appointments or outings today: Future appointments or outings:

Visitors: Concerns/Pain Levels/Emotions:

Date: Caregivers:

Wake/Sleep

1	2	3	4	5	6	7	8	9	10	11	12	1	2	3	4	5	6	7	8	9	10	11	12

Toilet	Time:						
	BM?						
	Change?						

Meals: Water: ⬡⬡⬡⬡⬡⬡⬡   Shower/Wash

Breakfast	AM snack	Lunch	PM snack	Dinner	Bedtime snack

Meds: ☐   ☐   ☐   ☐   ☐   ☐

Vitals:

Time	Blood pressure	Pulse	oxygen	Blood sugar		
	/					
	/					
	/					

Appointments or outings today: Future appointments or outings:

Visitors: Concerns/Pain Levels/Emotions:

Date: Caregivers:

Wake/Sleep

1	2	3	4	5	6	7	8	9	10	11	12	1	2	3	4	5	6	7	8	9	10	11	12

Toilet	Time:						
	BM?						
	Change?						

Meals: Water: ⬡⬡⬡⬡⬡⬡⬡⬡   Shower/Wash

Breakfast	AM snack	Lunch	PM snack	Dinner	Bedtime snack

Meds: ☐   ☐   ☐   ☐   ☐   ☐

Vitals:

Time	Blood pressure	Pulse	oxygen	Blood sugar		
	/					
	/					
	/					

Appointments or outings today: Future appointments or outings:

Visitors: Concerns/Pain Levels/Emotions:

General Notes/Additional Information

Date: **Caregivers:**

Wake/Sleep

1	2	3	4	5	6	7	8	9	10	11	12	1	2	3	4	5	6	7	8	9	10	11	12

Toilet	Time:						
	BM?						
	Change?						

Meals: **Water:** ◊◊◊◊◊◊◊   **Shower/Wash**

Breakfast	AM snack	Lunch	PM snack	Dinner	Bedtime snack

Meds: ☐   ☐   ☐   ☐   ☐   ☐

Vitals:

Time	Blood pressure	Pulse	oxygen	Blood sugar		
	/					
	/					
	/					

Appointments or outings today: **Future appointments or outings:**

Visitors: **Concerns/Pain Levels/Emotions:**

Date: Caregivers:

Wake/Sleep

1	2	3	4	5	6	7	8	9	10	11	12	1	2	3	4	5	6	7	8	9	10	11	12

Toilet	Time:						
	BM?						
	Change?						

Meals: Water: ◌◌◌◌◌◌◌   Shower/Wash

Breakfast	AM snack	Lunch	PM snack	Dinner	Bedtime snack

Meds: ☐   ☐   ☐   ☐   ☐   ☐

Vitals:

Time	Blood pressure	Pulse	oxygen	Blood sugar		
	/					
	/					
	/					

Appointments or outings today: Future appointments or outings:

Visitors: Concerns/Pain Levels/Emotions:

Date: Caregivers:

Wake/Sleep

1	2	3	4	5	6	7	8	9	10	11	12	1	2	3	4	5	6	7	8	9	10	11	12

Toilet	Time:						
	BM?						
	Change?						

Meals: Water: ⬠⬠⬠⬠⬠⬠⬠   Shower/Wash

Breakfast	AM snack	Lunch	PM snack	Dinner	Bedtime snack

Meds: ☐   ☐   ☐   ☐   ☐   ☐

Vitals:

Time	Blood pressure	Pulse	oxygen	Blood sugar		
	/					
	/					
	/					

Appointments or outings today: Future appointments or outings:

Visitors: Concerns/Pain Levels/Emotions:

Date: Caregivers:

Wake/Sleep

1	2	3	4	5	6	7	8	9	10	11	12	1	2	3	4	5	6	7	8	9	10	11	12

Toilet

Time:						
BM?						
Change?						

Meals: Water: ◊◊◊◊◊◊◊   Shower/Wash

Breakfast	AM snack	Lunch	PM snack	Dinner	Bedtime snack

Meds: ☐   ☐   ☐   ☐   ☐   ☐

Vitals:

Time	Blood pressure	Pulse	oxygen	Blood sugar		
	/					
	/					
	/					

Appointments or outings today: Future appointments or outings:

Visitors: Concerns/Pain Levels/Emotions:

Date: **Caregivers:**

Wake/Sleep

1	2	3	4	5	6	7	8	9	10	11	12	1	2	3	4	5	6	7	8	9	10	11	12

Toilet

Time:						
BM?						
Change?						

Meals: Water: ⬭⬭⬭⬭⬭⬭⬭   Shower/Wash

Breakfast	AM snack	Lunch	PM snack	Dinner	Bedtime snack

Meds: ☐   ☐   ☐   ☐   ☐   ☐

Vitals:

Time	Blood pressure	Pulse	oxygen	Blood sugar		
	/					
	/					
	/					

Appointments or outings today: Future appointments or outings:

Visitors: Concerns/Pain Levels/Emotions:

Date: Caregivers:

Wake/Sleep

1	2	3	4	5	6	7	8	9	10	11	12	1	2	3	4	5	6	7	8	9	10	11	12

Toilet

Time:						
BM?						
Change?						

Meals: Water: ◊◊◊◊◊◊◊◊   Shower/Wash

Breakfast	AM snack	Lunch	PM snack	Dinner	Bedtime snack

Meds: ☐   ☐   ☐   ☐   ☐   ☐

Vitals:

Time	Blood pressure	Pulse	oxygen	Blood sugar		
	/					
	/					
	/					

Appointments or outings today: Future appointments or outings:

Visitors: Concerns/Pain Levels/Emotions:

Date: Caregivers:

Wake/Sleep

1	2	3	4	5	6	7	8	9	10	11	12	1	2	3	4	5	6	7	8	9	10	11	12

Toilet	Time:						
	BM?						
	Change?						

Meals: Water: ◊◊◊◊◊◊◊   Shower/Wash

Breakfast	AM snack	Lunch	PM snack	Dinner	Bedtime snack

Meds: ☐   ☐   ☐   ☐   ☐   ☐

Vitals:

Time	Blood pressure	Pulse	oxygen	Blood sugar		
	/					
	/					
	/					

Appointments or outings today: Future appointments or outings:

Visitors: Concerns/Pain Levels/Emotions:

General Notes/Additional Information

Date: **Caregivers:**

Wake/Sleep

1	2	3	4	5	6	7	8	9	10	11	12	1	2	3	4	5	6	7	8	9	10	11	12

Toilet

Time:						
BM?						
Change?						

Meals: Water: ⬡⬡⬡⬡⬡⬡⬡   Shower/Wash

Breakfast	AM snack	Lunch	PM snack	Dinner	Bedtime snack

Meds: ☐   ☐   ☐   ☐   ☐   ☐

Vitals:

Time	Blood pressure	Pulse	oxygen	Blood sugar		
	/					
	/					
	/					

Appointments or outings today: Future appointments or outings:

Visitors: Concerns/Pain Levels/Emotions:

Date: Caregivers:

Wake/Sleep

1	2	3	4	5	6	7	8	9	10	11	12	1	2	3	4	5	6	7	8	9	10	11	12

Toilet	Time:							
	BM?							
	Change?							

Meals: Water: ◊◊◊◊◊◊◊   Shower/Wash

Breakfast	AM snack	Lunch	PM snack	Dinner	Bedtime snack

Meds: ☐   ☐   ☐   ☐   ☐   ☐

Vitals:

Time	Blood pressure	Pulse	oxygen	Blood sugar		
	/					
	/					
	/					

Appointments or outings today: Future appointments or outings:

Visitors: Concerns/Pain Levels/Emotions:

Date: Caregivers:

Wake/Sleep

1	2	3	4	5	6	7	8	9	10	11	12	1	2	3	4	5	6	7	8	9	10	11	12

Toilet	Time:							
	BM?							
	Change?							

Meals: Water: ◊◊◊◊◊◊◊◊   Shower/Wash

Breakfast	AM snack	Lunch	PM snack	Dinner	Bedtime snack

Meds: ☐   ☐   ☐   ☐   ☐   ☐

Vitals:

Time	Blood pressure	Pulse	oxygen	Blood sugar		
	/					
	/					
	/					

Appointments or outings today: Future appointments or outings:

Visitors: Concerns/Pain Levels/Emotions:

Date: Caregivers:

Wake/Sleep

1	2	3	4	5	6	7	8	9	10	11	12	1	2	3	4	5	6	7	8	9	10	11	12

Toilet	Time:						
	BM?						
	Change?						

Meals: Water: ◯◯◯◯◯◯◯◯   Shower/Wash

Breakfast	AM snack	Lunch	PM snack	Dinner	Bedtime snack

Meds: ☐   ☐   ☐   ☐   ☐   ☐

Vitals:

Time	Blood pressure	Pulse	oxygen	Blood sugar		
	/					
	/					
	/					

Appointments or outings today: Future appointments or outings:

Visitors: Concerns/Pain Levels/Emotions:

Date: Caregivers:

Wake/Sleep

1	2	3	4	5	6	7	8	9	10	11	12	1	2	3	4	5	6	7	8	9	10	11	12

Toilet	Time:						
	BM?						
	Change?						

Meals: Water: ⬡⬡⬡⬡⬡⬡⬡⬡   Shower/Wash

Breakfast	AM snack	Lunch	PM snack	Dinner	Bedtime snack

Meds: ☐   ☐   ☐   ☐   ☐   ☐

Vitals:

Time	Blood pressure	Pulse	oxygen	Blood sugar		
	/					
	/					
	/					

Appointments or outings today: Future appointments or outings:

Visitors: Concerns/Pain Levels/Emotions:

Date: Caregivers:

Wake/Sleep

1	2	3	4	5	6	7	8	9	10	11	12	1	2	3	4	5	6	7	8	9	10	11	12

Toilet

Time:						
BM?						
Change?						

Meals: Water: ◊◊◊◊◊◊◊◊   Shower/Wash

Breakfast	AM snack	Lunch	PM snack	Dinner	Bedtime snack

Meds: ☐   ☐   ☐   ☐   ☐   ☐

Vitals:

Time	Blood pressure	Pulse	oxygen	Blood sugar		
	/					
	/					
	/					

Appointments or outings today: Future appointments or outings:

Visitors: Concerns/Pain Levels/Emotions:

Date: **Caregivers:**

Wake/Sleep

1	2	3	4	5	6	7	8	9	10	11	12	1	2	3	4	5	6	7	8	9	10	11	12

Toilet	Time:						
	BM?						
	Change?						

Meals: Water: ⬡⬡⬡⬡⬡⬡⬡   Shower/Wash

Breakfast	AM snack	Lunch	PM snack	Dinner	Bedtime snack

Meds: ☐   ☐   ☐   ☐   ☐   ☐

Vitals:

Time	Blood pressure	Pulse	oxygen	Blood sugar		
	/					
	/					
	/					

Appointments or outings today: Future appointments or outings:

Visitors: Concerns/Pain Levels/Emotions:

General Notes/Additional Information

Date: Caregivers:

Wake/Sleep

1	2	3	4	5	6	7	8	9	10	11	12	1	2	3	4	5	6	7	8	9	10	11	12

Toilet

Time:							
BM?							
Change?							

Meals: Water: ◊◊◊◊◊◊◊   Shower/Wash

Breakfast	AM snack	Lunch	PM snack	Dinner	Bedtime snack

Meds: ☐   ☐   ☐   ☐   ☐   ☐

Vitals:

Time	Blood pressure	Pulse	oxygen	Blood sugar		
	/					
	/					
	/					

Appointments or outings today: Future appointments or outings:

Visitors: Concerns/Pain Levels/Emotions:

Date: Caregivers:

Wake/Sleep

1	2	3	4	5	6	7	8	9	10	11	12	1	2	3	4	5	6	7	8	9	10	11	12

Toilet	Time:						
	BM?						
	Change?						

Meals: Water: ⬭⬭⬭⬭⬭⬭⬭   Shower/Wash

Breakfast	AM snack	Lunch	PM snack	Dinner	Bedtime snack

Meds: ☐   ☐   ☐   ☐   ☐   ☐

Vitals:

Time	Blood pressure	Pulse	oxygen	Blood sugar		
	/					
	/					
	/					

Appointments or outings today: Future appointments or outings:

Visitors: Concerns/Pain Levels/Emotions:

Date: Caregivers:

Wake/Sleep

1	2	3	4	5	6	7	8	9	10	11	12	1	2	3	4	5	6	7	8	9	10	11	12

Toilet	Time:						
	BM?						
	Change?						

Meals: Water: ⬭⬭⬭⬭⬭⬭⬭⬭   Shower/Wash

Breakfast	AM snack	Lunch	PM snack	Dinner	Bedtime snack

Meds: ☐   ☐   ☐   ☐   ☐   ☐

Vitals:

Time	Blood pressure	Pulse	oxygen	Blood sugar		
	/					
	/					
	/					

Appointments or outings today: Future appointments or outings:

Visitors: Concerns/Pain Levels/Emotions:

Date: **Caregivers:**

Wake/Sleep

1	2	3	4	5	6	7	8	9	10	11	12	1	2	3	4	5	6	7	8	9	10	11	12

Toilet

Time:						
BM?						
Change?						

Meals: Water: ⬭⬭⬭⬭⬭⬭⬭⬭   Shower/Wash

Breakfast	AM snack	Lunch	PM snack	Dinner	Bedtime snack

Meds: ☐   ☐   ☐   ☐   ☐   ☐

Vitals:

Time	Blood pressure	Pulse	oxygen	Blood sugar		
	/					
	/					
	/					

Appointments or outings today: Future appointments or outings:

Visitors: Concerns/Pain Levels/Emotions:

Date: Caregivers:

Wake/Sleep

1	2	3	4	5	6	7	8	9	10	11	12	1	2	3	4	5	6	7	8	9	10	11	12

Toilet	Time:						
	BM?						
	Change?						

Meals: Water: ◊◊◊◊◊◊◊ Shower/Wash

Breakfast	AM snack	Lunch	PM snack	Dinner	Bedtime snack

Meds: ☐ ☐ ☐ ☐ ☐ ☐

Vitals:

Time	Blood pressure	Pulse	oxygen	Blood sugar		
	/					
	/					
	/					

Appointments or outings today: Future appointments or outings:

Visitors: Concerns/Pain Levels/Emotions:

Date: Caregivers:

Wake/Sleep

1	2	3	4	5	6	7	8	9	10	11	12	1	2	3	4	5	6	7	8	9	10	11	12

Toilet	Time:							
	BM?							
	Change?							

Meals: Water: ⬡⬡⬡⬡⬡⬡⬡   Shower/Wash

Breakfast	AM snack	Lunch	PM snack	Dinner	Bedtime snack

Meds: ☐   ☐   ☐   ☐   ☐   ☐

Vitals:

Time	Blood pressure	Pulse	oxygen	Blood sugar		
	/					
	/					
	/					

Appointments or outings today: Future appointments or outings:

Visitors: Concerns/Pain Levels/Emotions:

Date: Caregivers:

Wake/Sleep

1	2	3	4	5	6	7	8	9	10	11	12	1	2	3	4	5	6	7	8	9	10	11	12

Toilet

Time:						
BM?						
Change?						

Meals: Water: ◊◊◊◊◊◊◊◊   Shower/Wash

Breakfast	AM snack	Lunch	PM snack	Dinner	Bedtime snack

Meds: ☐   ☐   ☐   ☐   ☐   ☐

Vitals:

Time	Blood pressure	Pulse	oxygen	Blood sugar		
	/					
	/					
	/					

Appointments or outings today: Future appointments or outings:

Visitors: Concerns/Pain Levels/Emotions:

General Notes/Additional Information

Date: Caregivers:

Wake/Sleep

1	2	3	4	5	6	7	8	9	10	11	12	1	2	3	4	5	6	7	8	9	10	11	12

Toilet	Time:						
	BM?						
	Change?						

Meals: Water: ⬠⬠⬠⬠⬠⬠⬠   Shower/Wash

Breakfast	AM snack	Lunch	PM snack	Dinner	Bedtime snack

Meds: ☐   ☐   ☐   ☐   ☐   ☐

Vitals:

Time	Blood pressure	Pulse	oxygen	Blood sugar		
	/					
	/					
	/					

Appointments or outings today: Future appointments or outings:

Visitors: Concerns/Pain Levels/Emotions:

Date: Caregivers:

Wake/Sleep

1	2	3	4	5	6	7	8	9	10	11	12	1	2	3	4	5	6	7	8	9	10	11	12

Toilet	Time:						
	BM?						
	Change?						

Meals: Water: ◊◊◊◊◊◊◊   Shower/Wash

Breakfast	AM snack	Lunch	PM snack	Dinner	Bedtime snack

Meds: ☐   ☐   ☐   ☐   ☐   ☐

Vitals:

Time	Blood pressure	Pulse	oxygen	Blood sugar		
	/					
	/					
	/					

Appointments or outings today: Future appointments or outings:

Visitors: Concerns/Pain Levels/Emotions:

Date: Caregivers:

Wake/Sleep

1	2	3	4	5	6	7	8	9	10	11	12	1	2	3	4	5	6	7	8	9	10	11	12

Toilet	Time:							
	BM?							
	Change?							

Meals: Water: ◊◊◊◊◊◊◊◊   Shower/Wash

Breakfast	AM snack	Lunch	PM snack	Dinner	Bedtime snack

Meds: ☐   ☐   ☐   ☐   ☐   ☐

Vitals:

Time	Blood pressure	Pulse	oxygen	Blood sugar		
	/					
	/					
	/					

Appointments or outings today: Future appointments or outings:

Visitors: Concerns/Pain Levels/Emotions:

Date: Caregivers:

Wake/Sleep

1	2	3	4	5	6	7	8	9	10	11	12	1	2	3	4	5	6	7	8	9	10	11	12

Toilet	Time:						
	BM?						
	Change?						

Meals: Water: ◊◊◊◊◊◊◊   Shower/Wash

Breakfast	AM snack	Lunch	PM snack	Dinner	Bedtime snack

Meds: ☐   ☐   ☐   ☐   ☐   ☐

Vitals:

Time	Blood pressure	Pulse	oxygen	Blood sugar		
	/					
	/					
	/					

Appointments or outings today: Future appointments or outings:

Visitors: Concerns/Pain Levels/Emotions:

Date: Caregivers:

Wake/Sleep

1	2	3	4	5	6	7	8	9	10	11	12	1	2	3	4	5	6	7	8	9	10	11	12

Toilet	Time:						
	BM?						
	Change?						

Meals: Water: ◊◊◊◊◊◊◊◊   Shower/Wash

Breakfast	AM snack	Lunch	PM snack	Dinner	Bedtime snack

Meds: ☐   ☐   ☐   ☐   ☐   ☐

Vitals:

Time	Blood pressure	Pulse	oxygen	Blood sugar		
	/					
	/					
	/					

Appointments or outings today: Future appointments or outings:

Visitors: Concerns/Pain Levels/Emotions:

Date: Caregivers:

Wake/Sleep

1	2	3	4	5	6	7	8	9	10	11	12	1	2	3	4	5	6	7	8	9	10	11	12

Toilet	Time:							
	BM?							
	Change?							

Meals: Water: ⬡⬡⬡⬡⬡⬡⬡ Shower/Wash

Breakfast	AM snack	Lunch	PM snack	Dinner	Bedtime snack

Meds: ☐ ☐ ☐ ☐ ☐ ☐

Vitals:

Time	Blood pressure	Pulse	oxygen	Blood sugar		
	/					
	/					
	/					

Appointments or outings today: Future appointments or outings:

Visitors: Concerns/Pain Levels/Emotions:

Date: **Caregivers:**

Wake/Sleep

1	2	3	4	5	6	7	8	9	10	11	12	1	2	3	4	5	6	7	8	9	10	11	12

Toilet

Time:						
BM?						
Change?						

Meals: Water: ⬡⬡⬡⬡⬡⬡⬡⬡   Shower/Wash

Breakfast	AM snack	Lunch	PM snack	Dinner	Bedtime snack

Meds: ☐   ☐   ☐   ☐   ☐   ☐

Vitals:

Time	Blood pressure	Pulse	oxygen	Blood sugar		
	/					
	/					
	/					

Appointments or outings today: Future appointments or outings:

Visitors: Concerns/Pain Levels/Emotions:

General Notes/Additional Information

Date: Caregivers:

Wake/Sleep

1	2	3	4	5	6	7	8	9	10	11	12	1	2	3	4	5	6	7	8	9	10	11	12

Toilet

Time:						
BM?						
Change?						

Meals: Water: ◊◊◊◊◊◊◊   Shower/Wash

Breakfast	AM snack	Lunch	PM snack	Dinner	Bedtime snack

Meds: ☐   ☐   ☐   ☐   ☐   ☐

Vitals:

Time	Blood pressure	Pulse	oxygen	Blood sugar		
	/					
	/					
	/					

Appointments or outings today: Future appointments or outings:

Visitors: Concerns/Pain Levels/Emotions:

Date: Caregivers:

Wake/Sleep

1	2	3	4	5	6	7	8	9	10	11	12	1	2	3	4	5	6	7	8	9	10	11	12

Toilet	Time:							
	BM?							
	Change?							

Meals: Water: ⬡⬡⬡⬡⬡⬡⬡   Shower/Wash

Breakfast	AM snack	Lunch	PM snack	Dinner	Bedtime snack

Meds: ☐   ☐   ☐   ☐   ☐   ☐

Vitals:

Time	Blood pressure	Pulse	oxygen	Blood sugar		
	/					
	/					
	/					

Appointments or outings today: Future appointments or outings:

Visitors: Concerns/Pain Levels/Emotions:

Date: **Caregivers:**

Wake/Sleep

1	2	3	4	5	6	7	8	9	10	11	12	1	2	3	4	5	6	7	8	9	10	11	12

Toilet

Time:						
BM?						
Change?						

Meals: **Water:** ⬭⬭⬭⬭⬭⬭⬭⬭   **Shower/Wash**

Breakfast	AM snack	Lunch	PM snack	Dinner	Bedtime snack

Meds: ☐   ☐   ☐   ☐   ☐   ☐

Vitals:

Time	Blood pressure	Pulse	oxygen	Blood sugar		
	/					
	/					
	/					

Appointments or outings today: **Future appointments or outings:**

Visitors: **Concerns/Pain Levels/Emotions:**

Date: **Caregivers:**

Wake/Sleep

1	2	3	4	5	6	7	8	9	10	11	12	1	2	3	4	5	6	7	8	9	10	11	12

Toilet	Time:						
	BM?						
	Change?						

Meals: Water: ◊◊◊◊◊◊◊   Shower/Wash

Breakfast	AM snack	Lunch	PM snack	Dinner	Bedtime snack

Meds: ☐   ☐   ☐   ☐   ☐   ☐

Vitals:

Time	Blood pressure	Pulse	oxygen	Blood sugar		
	/					
	/					
	/					

Appointments or outings today: Future appointments or outings:

Visitors: Concerns/Pain Levels/Emotions:

Date: Caregivers:

Wake/Sleep

1	2	3	4	5	6	7	8	9	10	11	12	1	2	3	4	5	6	7	8	9	10	11	12

Toilet	Time:						
	BM?						
	Change?						

Meals: Water: ◊◊◊◊◊◊◊   Shower/Wash

Breakfast	AM snack	Lunch	PM snack	Dinner	Bedtime snack

Meds: ☐   ☐   ☐   ☐   ☐   ☐

Vitals:

Time	Blood pressure	Pulse	oxygen	Blood sugar		
	/					
	/					
	/					

Appointments or outings today: Future appointments or outings:

Visitors: Concerns/Pain Levels/Emotions:

Date: Caregivers:

Wake/Sleep

1	2	3	4	5	6	7	8	9	10	11	12	1	2	3	4	5	6	7	8	9	10	11	12

Toilet

Time:						
BM?						
Change?						

Meals: Water: ⬭⬭⬭⬭⬭⬭⬭   Shower/Wash

Breakfast	AM snack	Lunch	PM snack	Dinner	Bedtime snack

Meds: ☐   ☐   ☐   ☐   ☐   ☐

Vitals:

Time	Blood pressure	Pulse	oxygen	Blood sugar		
	/					
	/					
	/					

Appointments or outings today: Future appointments or outings:

Visitors: Concerns/Pain Levels/Emotions:

Date: Caregivers:

Wake/Sleep

1	2	3	4	5	6	7	8	9	10	11	12	1	2	3	4	5	6	7	8	9	10	11	12

Toilet	Time:							
	BM?							
	Change?							

Meals: Water: ⬡⬡⬡⬡⬡⬡⬡   Shower/Wash

Breakfast	AM snack	Lunch	PM snack	Dinner	Bedtime snack

Meds: ☐   ☐   ☐   ☐   ☐   ☐

Vitals:

Time	Blood pressure	Pulse	oxygen	Blood sugar		
	/					
	/					
	/					

Appointments or outings today: Future appointments or outings:

Visitors: Concerns/Pain Levels/Emotions:

General Notes/Additional Information

Date: Caregivers:

Wake/Sleep

1	2	3	4	5	6	7	8	9	10	11	12	1	2	3	4	5	6	7	8	9	10	11	12

Toilet

Time:						
BM?						
Change?						

Meals: Water: ◊◊◊◊◊◊◊   Shower/Wash

Breakfast	AM snack	Lunch	PM snack	Dinner	Bedtime snack

Meds: ☐   ☐   ☐   ☐   ☐   ☐

Vitals:

Time	Blood pressure	Pulse	oxygen	Blood sugar		
	/					
	/					
	/					

Appointments or outings today: Future appointments or outings:

Visitors: Concerns/Pain Levels/Emotions:

Date: Caregivers:

Wake/Sleep

1	2	3	4	5	6	7	8	9	10	11	12	1	2	3	4	5	6	7	8	9	10	11	12

Toilet

Time:							
BM?							
Change?							

Meals: Water: ⬭⬭⬭⬭⬭⬭⬭   Shower/Wash

Breakfast	AM snack	Lunch	PM snack	Dinner	Bedtime snack

Meds: ☐   ☐   ☐   ☐   ☐   ☐

Vitals:

Time	Blood pressure	Pulse	oxygen	Blood sugar		
	/					
	/					
	/					

Appointments or outings today: Future appointments or outings:

Visitors: Concerns/Pain Levels/Emotions:

Date: Caregivers:

Wake/Sleep

1	2	3	4	5	6	7	8	9	10	11	12	1	2	3	4	5	6	7	8	9	10	11	12

Toilet	Time:							
	BM?							
	Change?							

Meals: Water: ⬭⬭⬭⬭⬭⬭⬭⬭   Shower/Wash

Breakfast	AM snack	Lunch	PM snack	Dinner	Bedtime snack

Meds: ☐ ☐ ☐ ☐ ☐ ☐

Vitals:

Time	Blood pressure	Pulse	oxygen	Blood sugar		
	/					
	/					
	/					

Appointments or outings today: Future appointments or outings:

Visitors: Concerns/Pain Levels/Emotions:

Date: Caregivers:

Wake/Sleep

1	2	3	4	5	6	7	8	9	10	11	12	1	2	3	4	5	6	7	8	9	10	11	12

Toilet	Time:						
	BM?						
	Change?						

Meals: Water: ◊◊◊◊◊◊◊   Shower/Wash

Breakfast	AM snack	Lunch	PM snack	Dinner	Bedtime snack

Meds: ☐   ☐   ☐   ☐   ☐   ☐

Vitals:

Time	Blood pressure	Pulse	oxygen	Blood sugar		
	/					
	/					
	/					

Appointments or outings today: Future appointments or outings:

Visitors: Concerns/Pain Levels/Emotions:

Date: Caregivers:

Wake/Sleep

1	2	3	4	5	6	7	8	9	10	11	12	1	2	3	4	5	6	7	8	9	10	11	12

Toilet	Time:						
	BM?						
	Change?						

Meals: Water: ⬦⬦⬦⬦⬦⬦⬦   Shower/Wash

Breakfast	AM snack	Lunch	PM snack	Dinner	Bedtime snack

Meds: ☐   ☐   ☐   ☐   ☐   ☐

Vitals:

Time	Blood pressure	Pulse	oxygen	Blood sugar		
	/					
	/					
	/					

Appointments or outings today: Future appointments or outings:

Visitors: Concerns/Pain Levels/Emotions:

Date: Caregivers:

Wake/Sleep

1	2	3	4	5	6	7	8	9	10	11	12	1	2	3	4	5	6	7	8	9	10	11	12

Toilet

Time:						
BM?						
Change?						

Meals: Water: ⬡⬡⬡⬡⬡⬡⬡   Shower/Wash

Breakfast	AM snack	Lunch	PM snack	Dinner	Bedtime snack

Meds: ☐   ☐   ☐   ☐   ☐   ☐

Vitals:

Time	Blood pressure	Pulse	oxygen	Blood sugar		
	/					
	/					
	/					

Appointments or outings today: Future appointments or outings:

Visitors: Concerns/Pain Levels/Emotions:

Date: Caregivers:

Wake/Sleep

1	2	3	4	5	6	7	8	9	10	11	12	1	2	3	4	5	6	7	8	9	10	11	12

Toilet	Time:							
	BM?							
	Change?							

Meals: Water: ⬡⬡⬡⬡⬡⬡⬡⬡   Shower/Wash

Breakfast	AM snack	Lunch	PM snack	Dinner	Bedtime snack

Meds: ☐   ☐   ☐   ☐   ☐   ☐

Vitals:

Time	Blood pressure	Pulse	oxygen	Blood sugar		
	/					
	/					
	/					

Appointments or outings today: Future appointments or outings:

Visitors: Concerns/Pain Levels/Emotions:

General Notes/Additional Information

Date: Caregivers:

Wake/Sleep

1	2	3	4	5	6	7	8	9	10	11	12	1	2	3	4	5	6	7	8	9	10	11	12

Toilet	Time:						
	BM?						
	Change?						

Meals: Water: ⬡⬡⬡⬡⬡⬡⬡ Shower/Wash

Breakfast	AM snack	Lunch	PM snack	Dinner	Bedtime snack

Meds: ☐ ☐ ☐ ☐ ☐ ☐

Vitals:

Time	Blood pressure	Pulse	oxygen	Blood sugar		
	/					
	/					
	/					

Appointments or outings today: Future appointments or outings:

Visitors: Concerns/Pain Levels/Emotions:

Date: Caregivers:

Wake/Sleep

1	2	3	4	5	6	7	8	9	10	11	12	1	2	3	4	5	6	7	8	9	10	11	12

Toilet

Time:						
BM?						
Change?						

Meals: Water: ⬭⬭⬭⬭⬭⬭⬭   Shower/Wash

Breakfast	AM snack	Lunch	PM snack	Dinner	Bedtime snack

Meds: ☐   ☐   ☐   ☐   ☐   ☐

Vitals:

Time	Blood pressure	Pulse	oxygen	Blood sugar		
	/					
	/					
	/					

Appointments or outings today: Future appointments or outings:

Visitors: Concerns/Pain Levels/Emotions:

Date: **Caregivers:**

Wake/Sleep

1	2	3	4	5	6	7	8	9	10	11	12	1	2	3	4	5	6	7	8	9	10	11	12

Toilet	Time:							
	BM?							
	Change?							

Meals: **Water:** ⬡⬡⬡⬡⬡⬡⬡⬡   **Shower/Wash**

Breakfast	AM snack	Lunch	PM snack	Dinner	Bedtime snack

Meds: ☐   ☐   ☐   ☐   ☐   ☐

Vitals:

Time	Blood pressure	Pulse	oxygen	Blood sugar		
	/					
	/					
	/					

Appointments or outings today: **Future appointments or outings:**

Visitors: **Concerns/Pain Levels/Emotions:**

Date: Caregivers:

Wake/Sleep

1	2	3	4	5	6	7	8	9	10	11	12	1	2	3	4	5	6	7	8	9	10	11	12

Toilet	Time:						
	BM?						
	Change?						

Meals: Water: ⬡⬡⬡⬡⬡⬡⬡   Shower/Wash

Breakfast	AM snack	Lunch	PM snack	Dinner	Bedtime snack

Meds: ☐   ☐   ☐   ☐   ☐   ☐

Vitals:

Time	Blood pressure	Pulse	oxygen	Blood sugar		
	/					
	/					
	/					

Appointments or outings today: Future appointments or outings:

Visitors: Concerns/Pain Levels/Emotions:

Date: _____   Caregivers: _____

Wake/Sleep

1	2	3	4	5	6	7	8	9	10	11	12	1	2	3	4	5	6	7	8	9	10	11	12

Toilet	Time:						
	BM?						
	Change?						

Meals: Water: ⬡⬡⬡⬡⬡⬡⬡   Shower/Wash

Breakfast	AM snack	Lunch	PM snack	Dinner	Bedtime snack

Meds: ☐   ☐   ☐   ☐   ☐   ☐

Vitals:

Time	Blood pressure	Pulse	oxygen	Blood sugar		
	/					
	/					
	/					

Appointments or outings today: Future appointments or outings:

Visitors: Concerns/Pain Levels/Emotions:

Date: Caregivers:

Wake/Sleep

1	2	3	4	5	6	7	8	9	10	11	12	1	2	3	4	5	6	7	8	9	10	11	12

Toilet

Time:						
BM?						
Change?						

Meals: Water: ⬭⬭⬭⬭⬭⬭⬭   Shower/Wash

Breakfast	AM snack	Lunch	PM snack	Dinner	Bedtime snack

Meds: ☐   ☐   ☐   ☐   ☐   ☐

Vitals:

Time	Blood pressure	Pulse	oxygen	Blood sugar		
	/					
	/					
	/					

Appointments or outings today: Future appointments or outings:

Visitors: Concerns/Pain Levels/Emotions:

Date: Caregivers:

Wake/Sleep

1	2	3	4	5	6	7	8	9	10	11	12	1	2	3	4	5	6	7	8	9	10	11	12

Toilet

Time:							
BM?							
Change?							

Meals: Water: ◊◊◊◊◊◊◊◊   Shower/Wash

Breakfast	AM snack	Lunch	PM snack	Dinner	Bedtime snack

Meds: ☐   ☐   ☐   ☐   ☐   ☐

Vitals:

Time	Blood pressure	Pulse	oxygen	Blood sugar		
	/					
	/					
	/					

Appointments or outings today: Future appointments or outings:

Visitors: Concerns/Pain Levels/Emotions:

General Notes/Additional Information

Date: Caregivers:

Wake/Sleep

1	2	3	4	5	6	7	8	9	10	11	12	1	2	3	4	5	6	7	8	9	10	11	12

Toilet	Time:						
	BM?						
	Change?						

Meals: Water: ◊◊◊◊◊◊◊   Shower/Wash

Breakfast	AM snack	Lunch	PM snack	Dinner	Bedtime snack

Meds: ☐   ☐   ☐   ☐   ☐   ☐

Vitals:

Time	Blood pressure	Pulse	oxygen	Blood sugar		
	/					
	/					
	/					

Appointments or outings today: Future appointments or outings:

Visitors: Concerns/Pain Levels/Emotions:

Date: Caregivers:

Wake/Sleep

1	2	3	4	5	6	7	8	9	10	11	12	1	2	3	4	5	6	7	8	9	10	11	12

Toilet

Time:							
BM?							
Change?							

Meals: Water: ⬭⬭⬭⬭⬭⬭⬭   Shower/Wash

Breakfast	AM snack	Lunch	PM snack	Dinner	Bedtime snack

Meds: ☐   ☐   ☐   ☐   ☐   ☐

Vitals:

Time	Blood pressure	Pulse	oxygen	Blood sugar		
	/					
	/					
	/					

Appointments or outings today: Future appointments or outings:

Visitors: Concerns/Pain Levels/Emotions:

Date: Caregivers:

Wake/Sleep

1	2	3	4	5	6	7	8	9	10	11	12	1	2	3	4	5	6	7	8	9	10	11	12

Toilet
Time:						
BM?						
Change?						

Meals: Water: ⬡⬡⬡⬡⬡⬡⬡⬡   Shower/Wash

Breakfast	AM snack	Lunch	PM snack	Dinner	Bedtime snack

Meds: ☐   ☐   ☐   ☐   ☐   ☐

Vitals:

Time	Blood pressure	Pulse	oxygen	Blood sugar		
	/					
	/					
	/					

Appointments or outings today: Future appointments or outings:

Visitors: Concerns/Pain Levels/Emotions:

Date: Caregivers:

Wake/Sleep

1	2	3	4	5	6	7	8	9	10	11	12	1	2	3	4	5	6	7	8	9	10	11	12

Toilet	Time:						
	BM?						
	Change?						

Meals: Water: ⬭⬭⬭⬭⬭⬭⬭   Shower/Wash

Breakfast	AM snack	Lunch	PM snack	Dinner	Bedtime snack

Meds: ☐   ☐   ☐   ☐   ☐   ☐

Vitals:

Time	Blood pressure	Pulse	oxygen	Blood sugar		
	/					
	/					
	/					

Appointments or outings today: Future appointments or outings:

Visitors: Concerns/Pain Levels/Emotions:

Date: Caregivers:

Wake/Sleep

1	2	3	4	5	6	7	8	9	10	11	12	1	2	3	4	5	6	7	8	9	10	11	12

Toilet	Time:						
	BM?						
	Change?						

Meals: Water: ◊◊◊◊◊◊◊   Shower/Wash

Breakfast	AM snack	Lunch	PM snack	Dinner	Bedtime snack

Meds: ☐   ☐   ☐   ☐   ☐   ☐

Vitals:

Time	Blood pressure	Pulse	oxygen	Blood sugar		
	/					
	/					
	/					

Appointments or outings today: Future appointments or outings:

Visitors: Concerns/Pain Levels/Emotions:

Date: Caregivers:

Wake/Sleep

1	2	3	4	5	6	7	8	9	10	11	12	1	2	3	4	5	6	7	8	9	10	11	12

Toilet

Time:							
BM?							
Change?							

Meals: Water: ⬡⬡⬡⬡⬡⬡⬡   Shower/Wash

Breakfast	AM snack	Lunch	PM snack	Dinner	Bedtime snack

Meds: ☐   ☐   ☐   ☐   ☐   ☐

Vitals:

Time	Blood pressure	Pulse	oxygen	Blood sugar		
	/					
	/					
	/					

Appointments or outings today: Future appointments or outings:

Visitors: Concerns/Pain Levels/Emotions:

Date: **Caregivers:**

Wake/Sleep

1	2	3	4	5	6	7	8	9	10	11	12	1	2	3	4	5	6	7	8	9	10	11	12

Toilet	Time:						
	BM?						
	Change?						

Meals: Water: ◇◇◇◇◇◇◇◇   Shower/Wash

Breakfast	AM snack	Lunch	PM snack	Dinner	Bedtime snack

Meds: ☐   ☐   ☐   ☐   ☐   ☐

Vitals:

Time	Blood pressure	Pulse	oxygen	Blood sugar		
	/					
	/					
	/					

Appointments or outings today: Future appointments or outings:

Visitors: Concerns/Pain Levels/Emotions:

General Notes/Additional Information

Date:

Caregivers:

Wake/Sleep

1	2	3	4	5	6	7	8	9	10	11	12	1	2	3	4	5	6	7	8	9	10	11	12

Toilet	Time:						
	BM?						
	Change?						

Meals: Water: ◊◊◊◊◊◊◊◊   Shower/Wash

Breakfast	AM snack	Lunch	PM snack	Dinner	Bedtime snack

Meds: ☐   ☐   ☐   ☐   ☐   ☐

Vitals:

Time	Blood pressure	Pulse	oxygen	Blood sugar		
	/					
	/					
	/					

Appointments or outings today: Future appointments or outings:

Visitors: Concerns/Pain Levels/Emotions:

Date: Caregivers:

Wake/Sleep

1	2	3	4	5	6	7	8	9	10	11	12	1	2	3	4	5	6	7	8	9	10	11	12

Toilet

Time:							
BM?							
Change?							

Meals: Water: ⬭⬭⬭⬭⬭⬭⬭   Shower/Wash

Breakfast	AM snack	Lunch	PM snack	Dinner	Bedtime snack

Meds: ☐   ☐   ☐   ☐   ☐   ☐

Vitals:

Time	Blood pressure	Pulse	oxygen	Blood sugar		
	/					
	/					
	/					

Appointments or outings today: Future appointments or outings:

Visitors: Concerns/Pain Levels/Emotions:

Date: Caregivers:

Wake/Sleep

1	2	3	4	5	6	7	8	9	10	11	12	1	2	3	4	5	6	7	8	9	10	11	12

Toilet

Time:							
BM?							
Change?							

Meals: Water: ⬡⬡⬡⬡⬡⬡⬡⬡   Shower/Wash

Breakfast	AM snack	Lunch	PM snack	Dinner	Bedtime snack

Meds: ☐   ☐   ☐   ☐   ☐   ☐

Vitals:

Time	Blood pressure	Pulse	oxygen	Blood sugar		
	/					
	/					
	/					

Appointments or outings today: Future appointments or outings:

Visitors: Concerns/Pain Levels/Emotions:

Date: Caregivers:

Wake/Sleep

1	2	3	4	5	6	7	8	9	10	11	12	1	2	3	4	5	6	7	8	9	10	11	12

Toilet

Time:						
BM?						
Change?						

Meals: Water: ◊◊◊◊◊◊◊◊   Shower/Wash

Breakfast	AM snack	Lunch	PM snack	Dinner	Bedtime snack

Meds: ☐   ☐   ☐   ☐   ☐   ☐

Vitals:

Time	Blood pressure	Pulse	oxygen	Blood sugar		
	/					
	/					
	/					

Appointments or outings today: Future appointments or outings:

Visitors: Concerns/Pain Levels/Emotions:

Date: **Caregivers:**

Wake/Sleep

1	2	3	4	5	6	7	8	9	10	11	12	1	2	3	4	5	6	7	8	9	10	11	12

Toilet

Time:						
BM?						
Change?						

Meals: **Water:** ⬭⬭⬭⬭⬭⬭⬭   **Shower/Wash**

Breakfast	AM snack	Lunch	PM snack	Dinner	Bedtime snack

Meds: ☐   ☐   ☐   ☐   ☐   ☐

Vitals:

Time	Blood pressure	Pulse	oxygen	Blood sugar		
	/					
	/					
	/					

Appointments or outings today: **Future appointments or outings:**

Visitors: **Concerns/Pain Levels/Emotions:**

Date: Caregivers:

Wake/Sleep

1	2	3	4	5	6	7	8	9	10	11	12	1	2	3	4	5	6	7	8	9	10	11	12

Toilet

Time:						
BM?						
Change?						

Meals: Water: ◊◊◊◊◊◊◊   Shower/Wash

Breakfast	AM snack	Lunch	PM snack	Dinner	Bedtime snack

Meds: ☐   ☐   ☐   ☐   ☐   ☐

Vitals:

Time	Blood pressure	Pulse	oxygen	Blood sugar		
	/					
	/					
	/					

Appointments or outings today: Future appointments or outings:

Visitors: Concerns/Pain Levels/Emotions:

Date: Caregivers:

Wake/Sleep

1	2	3	4	5	6	7	8	9	10	11	12	1	2	3	4	5	6	7	8	9	10	11	12

Toilet	Time:						
	BM?						
	Change?						

Meals: Water: ⬡⬡⬡⬡⬡⬡⬡ Shower/Wash

Breakfast	AM snack	Lunch	PM snack	Dinner	Bedtime snack

Meds: ☐ ☐ ☐ ☐ ☐ ☐

Vitals:

Time	Blood pressure	Pulse	oxygen	Blood sugar		
	/					
	/					
	/					

Appointments or outings today: Future appointments or outings:

Visitors: Concerns/Pain Levels/Emotions:

General Notes/Additional Information

Date: _____   Caregivers: _____

Wake/Sleep

1	2	3	4	5	6	7	8	9	10	11	12	1	2	3	4	5	6	7	8	9	10	11	12

Toilet	Time:						
	BM?						
	Change?						

Meals: Water: ⬠⬠⬠⬠⬠⬠⬠   Shower/Wash

Breakfast	AM snack	Lunch	PM snack	Dinner	Bedtime snack

Meds: ☐   ☐   ☐   ☐   ☐   ☐

Vitals:

Time	Blood pressure	Pulse	oxygen	Blood sugar		
	/					
	/					
	/					

Appointments or outings today: Future appointments or outings:

Visitors: Concerns/Pain Levels/Emotions:

Date: Caregivers:

Wake/Sleep

1	2	3	4	5	6	7	8	9	10	11	12	1	2	3	4	5	6	7	8	9	10	11	12

Toilet

Time:						
BM?						
Change?						

Meals: Water: ⬡⬡⬡⬡⬡⬡⬡   Shower/Wash

Breakfast	AM snack	Lunch	PM snack	Dinner	Bedtime snack

Meds: ☐   ☐   ☐   ☐   ☐   ☐

Vitals:

Time	Blood pressure	Pulse	oxygen	Blood sugar		
	/					
	/					
	/					

Appointments or outings today: Future appointments or outings:

Visitors: Concerns/Pain Levels/Emotions:

Date: **Caregivers:**

Wake/Sleep

1	2	3	4	5	6	7	8	9	10	11	12	1	2	3	4	5	6	7	8	9	10	11	12

Toilet	Time:							
	BM?							
	Change?							

Meals: Water: ○○○○○○○○   Shower/Wash

Breakfast	AM snack	Lunch	PM snack	Dinner	Bedtime snack

Meds: ☐   ☐   ☐   ☐   ☐   ☐

Vitals:

Time	Blood pressure	Pulse	oxygen	Blood sugar		
	/					
	/					
	/					

Appointments or outings today: Future appointments or outings:

Visitors: Concerns/Pain Levels/Emotions:

Date: Caregivers:

Wake/Sleep

1	2	3	4	5	6	7	8	9	10	11	12	1	2	3	4	5	6	7	8	9	10	11	12

Toilet

Time:						
BM?						
Change?						

Meals: Water: ⬡⬡⬡⬡⬡⬡⬡   Shower/Wash

Breakfast	AM snack	Lunch	PM snack	Dinner	Bedtime snack

Meds: ☐   ☐   ☐   ☐   ☐   ☐

Vitals:

Time	Blood pressure	Pulse	oxygen	Blood sugar		
	/					
	/					
	/					

Appointments or outings today: Future appointments or outings:

Visitors: Concerns/Pain Levels/Emotions:

Date: Caregivers:

Wake/Sleep

1	2	3	4	5	6	7	8	9	10	11	12	1	2	3	4	5	6	7	8	9	10	11	12

Toilet	Time:						
	BM?						
	Change?						

Meals: Water: ◊◊◊◊◊◊◊   Shower/Wash

Breakfast	AM snack	Lunch	PM snack	Dinner	Bedtime snack

Meds: ☐   ☐   ☐   ☐   ☐   ☐

Vitals:

Time	Blood pressure	Pulse	oxygen	Blood sugar		
	/					
	/					
	/					

Appointments or outings today: Future appointments or outings:

Visitors: Concerns/Pain Levels/Emotions:

Date: Caregivers:

Wake/Sleep

1	2	3	4	5	6	7	8	9	10	11	12	1	2	3	4	5	6	7	8	9	10	11	12

Toilet

Time:							
BM?							
Change?							

Meals: Water: ⬡⬡⬡⬡⬡⬡⬡   Shower/Wash

Breakfast	AM snack	Lunch	PM snack	Dinner	Bedtime snack

Meds: ☐   ☐   ☐   ☐   ☐   ☐

Vitals:

Time	Blood pressure	Pulse	oxygen	Blood sugar		
	/					
	/					
	/					

Appointments or outings today: Future appointments or outings:

Visitors: Concerns/Pain Levels/Emotions:

Date: **Caregivers:**

Wake/Sleep

1	2	3	4	5	6	7	8	9	10	11	12	1	2	3	4	5	6	7	8	9	10	11	12

Toilet

Time:						
BM?						
Change?						

Meals: **Water:** ⬡⬡⬡⬡⬡⬡⬡⬡   **Shower/Wash**

Breakfast	AM snack	Lunch	PM snack	Dinner	Bedtime snack

Meds: ☐   ☐   ☐   ☐   ☐   ☐

Vitals:

Time	Blood pressure	Pulse	oxygen	Blood sugar		
	/					
	/					
	/					

Appointments or outings today: Future appointments or outings:

Visitors: Concerns/Pain Levels/Emotions:

General Notes/Additional Information

Date: Caregivers:

Wake/Sleep

1	2	3	4	5	6	7	8	9	10	11	12	1	2	3	4	5	6	7	8	9	10	11	12

Toilet	Time:						
	BM?						
	Change?						

Meals: Water: ◊◊◊◊◊◊◊   Shower/Wash

Breakfast	AM snack	Lunch	PM snack	Dinner	Bedtime snack

Meds: ☐   ☐   ☐   ☐   ☐   ☐

Vitals:

Time	Blood pressure	Pulse	oxygen	Blood sugar		
	/					
	/					
	/					

Appointments or outings today: Future appointments or outings:

Visitors: Concerns/Pain Levels/Emotions:

Date: Caregivers:

Wake/Sleep

1	2	3	4	5	6	7	8	9	10	11	12	1	2	3	4	5	6	7	8	9	10	11	12

Toilet

Time:							
BM?							
Change?							

Meals: Water: ◊◊◊◊◊◊◊◊   Shower/Wash

Breakfast	AM snack	Lunch	PM snack	Dinner	Bedtime snack

Meds: ☐   ☐   ☐   ☐   ☐   ☐

Vitals:

Time	Blood pressure	Pulse	oxygen	Blood sugar		
	/					
	/					
	/					

Appointments or outings today: Future appointments or outings:

Visitors: Concerns/Pain Levels/Emotions:

Date: Caregivers:

Wake/Sleep

1	2	3	4	5	6	7	8	9	10	11	12	1	2	3	4	5	6	7	8	9	10	11	12

Toilet	Time:						
	BM?						
	Change?						

Meals: Water: ⬡⬡⬡⬡⬡⬡⬡   Shower/Wash

Breakfast	AM snack	Lunch	PM snack	Dinner	Bedtime snack

Meds: ☐   ☐   ☐   ☐   ☐   ☐

Vitals:

Time	Blood pressure	Pulse	oxygen	Blood sugar		
	/					
	/					
	/					

Appointments or outings today: Future appointments or outings:

Visitors: Concerns/Pain Levels/Emotions:

Date: Caregivers:

Wake/Sleep

1	2	3	4	5	6	7	8	9	10	11	12	1	2	3	4	5	6	7	8	9	10	11	12

Toilet	Time:						
	BM?						
	Change?						

Meals: Water: ⟡⟡⟡⟡⟡⟡⟡   Shower/Wash

Breakfast	AM snack	Lunch	PM snack	Dinner	Bedtime snack

Meds: ☐   ☐   ☐   ☐   ☐   ☐

Vitals:

Time	Blood pressure	Pulse	oxygen	Blood sugar		
	/					
	/					
	/					

Appointments or outings today: Future appointments or outings:

Visitors: Concerns/Pain Levels/Emotions:

Date: Caregivers:

Wake/Sleep

1	2	3	4	5	6	7	8	9	10	11	12	1	2	3	4	5	6	7	8	9	10	11	12

Toilet	Time:						
	BM?						
	Change?						

Meals: Water: ◊◊◊◊◊◊◊   Shower/Wash

Breakfast	AM snack	Lunch	PM snack	Dinner	Bedtime snack

Meds: ☐   ☐   ☐   ☐   ☐   ☐

Vitals:

Time	Blood pressure	Pulse	oxygen	Blood sugar		
	/					
	/					
	/					

Appointments or outings today: Future appointments or outings:

Visitors: Concerns/Pain Levels/Emotions:

Date: Caregivers:

Wake/Sleep

1	2	3	4	5	6	7	8	9	10	11	12	1	2	3	4	5	6	7	8	9	10	11	12

Toilet

Time:							
BM?							
Change?							

Meals: Water: ⬭⬭⬭⬭⬭⬭⬭   Shower/Wash

Breakfast	AM snack	Lunch	PM snack	Dinner	Bedtime snack

Meds: ☐   ☐   ☐   ☐   ☐   ☐

Vitals:

Time	Blood pressure	Pulse	oxygen	Blood sugar		
	/					
	/					
	/					

Appointments or outings today: Future appointments or outings:

Visitors: Concerns/Pain Levels/Emotions:

Date: Caregivers:

Wake/Sleep

1	2	3	4	5	6	7	8	9	10	11	12	1	2	3	4	5	6	7	8	9	10	11	12

Toilet	Time:							
	BM?							
	Change?							

Meals: Water: ⬡⬡⬡⬡⬡⬡⬡⬡   Shower/Wash

Breakfast	AM snack	Lunch	PM snack	Dinner	Bedtime snack

Meds: ☐   ☐   ☐   ☐   ☐   ☐

Vitals:

Time	Blood pressure	Pulse	oxygen	Blood sugar		
	/					
	/					
	/					

Appointments or outings today: Future appointments or outings:

Visitors: Concerns/Pain Levels/Emotions:

General Notes/Additional Information

Date: **Caregivers:**

Wake/Sleep

1	2	3	4	5	6	7	8	9	10	11	12	1	2	3	4	5	6	7	8	9	10	11	12

Toilet	Time:						
	BM?						
	Change?						

Meals: **Water:** ⬡⬡⬡⬡⬡⬡⬡   **Shower/Wash**

Breakfast	AM snack	Lunch	PM snack	Dinner	Bedtime snack

Meds: ☐   ☐   ☐   ☐   ☐   ☐

Vitals:

Time	Blood pressure	Pulse	oxygen	Blood sugar		
	/					
	/					
	/					

Appointments or outings today: **Future appointments or outings:**

Visitors: **Concerns/Pain Levels/Emotions:**

Date: Caregivers:

Wake/Sleep

1	2	3	4	5	6	7	8	9	10	11	12	1	2	3	4	5	6	7	8	9	10	11	12

Toilet

Time:							
BM?							
Change?							

Meals: Water: ⬡⬡⬡⬡⬡⬡⬡   Shower/Wash

Breakfast	AM snack	Lunch	PM snack	Dinner	Bedtime snack

Meds: ☐   ☐   ☐   ☐   ☐   ☐

Vitals:

Time	Blood pressure	Pulse	oxygen	Blood sugar		
	/					
	/					
	/					

Appointments or outings today: Future appointments or outings:

Visitors: Concerns/Pain Levels/Emotions:

Date: Caregivers:

Wake/Sleep

1	2	3	4	5	6	7	8	9	10	11	12	1	2	3	4	5	6	7	8	9	10	11	12

Toilet	Time:						
	BM?						
	Change?						

Meals: Water: ⬠⬠⬠⬠⬠⬠⬠⬠   Shower/Wash

Breakfast	AM snack	Lunch	PM snack	Dinner	Bedtime snack

Meds: ☐   ☐   ☐   ☐   ☐   ☐

Vitals:

Time	Blood pressure	Pulse	oxygen	Blood sugar		
	/					
	/					
	/					

Appointments or outings today: Future appointments or outings:

Visitors: Concerns/Pain Levels/Emotions:

Date: Caregivers:

Wake/Sleep

1	2	3	4	5	6	7	8	9	10	11	12	1	2	3	4	5	6	7	8	9	10	11	12

Toilet

Time:						
BM?						
Change?						

Meals: Water: ⬭⬭⬭⬭⬭⬭⬭   Shower/Wash

Breakfast	AM snack	Lunch	PM snack	Dinner	Bedtime snack

Meds: ☐   ☐   ☐   ☐   ☐   ☐

Vitals:

Time	Blood pressure	Pulse	oxygen	Blood sugar		
	/					
	/					
	/					

Appointments or outings today: Future appointments or outings:

Visitors: Concerns/Pain Levels/Emotions:

Date: Caregivers:

Wake/Sleep

1	2	3	4	5	6	7	8	9	10	11	12	1	2	3	4	5	6	7	8	9	10	11	12

Toilet	Time:							
	BM?							
	Change?							

Meals: Water: ◊◊◊◊◊◊◊   Shower/Wash

Breakfast	AM snack	Lunch	PM snack	Dinner	Bedtime snack

Meds: ☐   ☐   ☐   ☐   ☐   ☐

Vitals:

Time	Blood pressure	Pulse	oxygen	Blood sugar		
	/					
	/					
	/					

Appointments or outings today: Future appointments or outings:

Visitors: Concerns/Pain Levels/Emotions:

Date: Caregivers:

Wake/Sleep

1	2	3	4	5	6	7	8	9	10	11	12	1	2	3	4	5	6	7	8	9	10	11	12

Toilet	Time:							
	BM?							
	Change?							

Meals: Water: ⚪⚪⚪⚪⚪⚪⚪   Shower/Wash

Breakfast	AM snack	Lunch	PM snack	Dinner	Bedtime snack

Meds: ☐   ☐   ☐   ☐   ☐   ☐

Vitals:

Time	Blood pressure	Pulse	oxygen	Blood sugar		
	/					
	/					
	/					

Appointments or outings today: Future appointments or outings:

Visitors: Concerns/Pain Levels/Emotions:

Date: Caregivers:

Wake/Sleep

1	2	3	4	5	6	7	8	9	10	11	12	1	2	3	4	5	6	7	8	9	10	11	12

Toilet

Time:						
BM?						
Change?						

Meals: Water: ◊◊◊◊◊◊◊◊   Shower/Wash

Breakfast	AM snack	Lunch	PM snack	Dinner	Bedtime snack

Meds: ☐   ☐   ☐   ☐   ☐   ☐

Vitals:

Time	Blood pressure	Pulse	oxygen	Blood sugar		
	/					
	/					
	/					

Appointments or outings today: Future appointments or outings:

Visitors: Concerns/Pain Levels/Emotions:

General Notes/Additional Information

Date: Caregivers:

Wake/Sleep

1	2	3	4	5	6	7	8	9	10	11	12	1	2	3	4	5	6	7	8	9	10	11	12

Toilet	Time:						
	BM?						
	Change?						

Meals: Water: ⬦⬦⬦⬦⬦⬦⬦   Shower/Wash

Breakfast	AM snack	Lunch	PM snack	Dinner	Bedtime snack

Meds: ☐   ☐   ☐   ☐   ☐   ☐

Vitals:

Time	Blood pressure	Pulse	oxygen	Blood sugar		
	/					
	/					
	/					

Appointments or outings today: Future appointments or outings:

Visitors: Concerns/Pain Levels/Emotions:

Date: Caregivers:

Wake/Sleep

1	2	3	4	5	6	7	8	9	10	11	12	1	2	3	4	5	6	7	8	9	10	11	12

Toilet

Time:						
BM?						
Change?						

Meals: Water: ⬡⬡⬡⬡⬡⬡⬡ Shower/Wash

Breakfast	AM snack	Lunch	PM snack	Dinner	Bedtime snack

Meds: ☐ ☐ ☐ ☐ ☐ ☐

Vitals:

Time	Blood pressure	Pulse	oxygen	Blood sugar		
	/					
	/					
	/					

Appointments or outings today: Future appointments or outings:

Visitors: Concerns/Pain Levels/Emotions:

Date: Caregivers:

Wake/Sleep

1	2	3	4	5	6	7	8	9	10	11	12	1	2	3	4	5	6	7	8	9	10	11	12

Toilet	Time:						
	BM?						
	Change?						

Meals: Water: ◊◊◊◊◊◊◊◊   Shower/Wash

Breakfast	AM snack	Lunch	PM snack	Dinner	Bedtime snack

Meds: ☐   ☐   ☐   ☐   ☐   ☐

Vitals:

Time	Blood pressure	Pulse	oxygen	Blood sugar		
	/					
	/					
	/					

Appointments or outings today: Future appointments or outings:

Visitors: Concerns/Pain Levels/Emotions:

Date: Caregivers:

Wake/Sleep

1	2	3	4	5	6	7	8	9	10	11	12	1	2	3	4	5	6	7	8	9	10	11	12

Toilet	Time:						
	BM?						
	Change?						

Meals: Water: ◊◊◊◊◊◊◊◊ Shower/Wash

Breakfast	AM snack	Lunch	PM snack	Dinner	Bedtime snack

Meds: ☐ ☐ ☐ ☐ ☐ ☐

Vitals:

Time	Blood pressure	Pulse	oxygen	Blood sugar		
	/					
	/					
	/					

Appointments or outings today: Future appointments or outings:

Visitors: Concerns/Pain Levels/Emotions:

Date: Caregivers:

Wake/Sleep

1	2	3	4	5	6	7	8	9	10	11	12	1	2	3	4	5	6	7	8	9	10	11	12

Toilet	Time:						
	BM?						
	Change?						

Meals: Water: ⬭⬭⬭⬭⬭⬭⬭   Shower/Wash

Breakfast	AM snack	Lunch	PM snack	Dinner	Bedtime snack

Meds: ☐   ☐   ☐   ☐   ☐   ☐

Vitals:

Time	Blood pressure	Pulse	oxygen	Blood sugar		
	/					
	/					
	/					

Appointments or outings today: Future appointments or outings:

Visitors: Concerns/Pain Levels/Emotions:

Date: Caregivers:

Wake/Sleep

1	2	3	4	5	6	7	8	9	10	11	12	1	2	3	4	5	6	7	8	9	10	11	12

Toilet

Time:						
BM?						
Change?						

Meals: Water: ⬭⬭⬭⬭⬭⬭⬭   Shower/Wash

Breakfast	AM snack	Lunch	PM snack	Dinner	Bedtime snack

Meds: ☐   ☐   ☐   ☐   ☐   ☐

Vitals:

Time	Blood pressure	Pulse	oxygen	Blood sugar		
	/					
	/					
	/					

Appointments or outings today: Future appointments or outings:

Visitors: Concerns/Pain Levels/Emotions:

Date: **Caregivers:**

Wake/Sleep

1	2	3	4	5	6	7	8	9	10	11	12	1	2	3	4	5	6	7	8	9	10	11	12

Toilet	Time:						
	BM?						
	Change?						

Meals: Water: ⬡⬡⬡⬡⬡⬡⬡⬡   Shower/Wash

Breakfast	AM snack	Lunch	PM snack	Dinner	Bedtime snack

Meds: ☐   ☐   ☐   ☐   ☐   ☐

Vitals:

Time	Blood pressure	Pulse	oxygen	Blood sugar		
	/					
	/					
	/					

Appointments or outings today: Future appointments or outings:

Visitors: Concerns/Pain Levels/Emotions:

General Notes/Additional Information

Date: Caregivers:

Wake/Sleep

1	2	3	4	5	6	7	8	9	10	11	12	1	2	3	4	5	6	7	8	9	10	11	12

Toilet	Time:						
	BM?						
	Change?						

Meals: Water: ◊◊◊◊◊◊◊   Shower/Wash

Breakfast	AM snack	Lunch	PM snack	Dinner	Bedtime snack

Meds: ☐   ☐   ☐   ☐   ☐   ☐

Vitals:

Time	Blood pressure	Pulse	oxygen	Blood sugar		
	/					
	/					
	/					

Appointments or outings today: Future appointments or outings:

Visitors: Concerns/Pain Levels/Emotions:

Date: Caregivers:

Wake/Sleep

1	2	3	4	5	6	7	8	9	10	11	12	1	2	3	4	5	6	7	8	9	10	11	12

Toilet

Time:							
BM?							
Change?							

Meals: Water: ⬠⬠⬠⬠⬠⬠⬠   Shower/Wash

Breakfast	AM snack	Lunch	PM snack	Dinner	Bedtime snack

Meds: ☐   ☐   ☐   ☐   ☐   ☐

Vitals:

Time	Blood pressure	Pulse	oxygen	Blood sugar		
	/					
	/					
	/					

Appointments or outings today: Future appointments or outings:

Visitors: Concerns/Pain Levels/Emotions:

Date: _____   Caregivers: _____

Wake/Sleep

1	2	3	4	5	6	7	8	9	10	11	12	1	2	3	4	5	6	7	8	9	10	11	12

Toilet	Time:						
	BM?						
	Change?						

Meals: Water: ⬦⬦⬦⬦⬦⬦⬦⬦   Shower/Wash

Breakfast	AM snack	Lunch	PM snack	Dinner	Bedtime snack

Meds: ☐   ☐   ☐   ☐   ☐   ☐

Vitals:

Time	Blood pressure	Pulse	oxygen	Blood sugar		
	/					
	/					
	/					

Appointments or outings today: Future appointments or outings:

Visitors: Concerns/Pain Levels/Emotions:

Date: Caregivers:

Wake/Sleep

1	2	3	4	5	6	7	8	9	10	11	12	1	2	3	4	5	6	7	8	9	10	11	12

Toilet

Time:							
BM?							
Change?							

Meals: Water: ⬠⬠⬠⬠⬠⬠⬠   Shower/Wash

Breakfast	AM snack	Lunch	PM snack	Dinner	Bedtime snack

Meds: ☐   ☐   ☐   ☐   ☐   ☐

Vitals:

Time	Blood pressure	Pulse	oxygen	Blood sugar		
	/					
	/					
	/					

Appointments or outings today: Future appointments or outings:

Visitors: Concerns/Pain Levels/Emotions:

Date: Caregivers:

Wake/Sleep

1	2	3	4	5	6	7	8	9	10	11	12	1	2	3	4	5	6	7	8	9	10	11	12

Toilet	Time:						
	BM?						
	Change?						

Meals: Water: ◊◊◊◊◊◊◊   Shower/Wash

Breakfast	AM snack	Lunch	PM snack	Dinner	Bedtime snack

Meds: ☐   ☐   ☐   ☐   ☐   ☐

Vitals:

Time	Blood pressure	Pulse	oxygen	Blood sugar		
	/					
	/					
	/					

Appointments or outings today: Future appointments or outings:

Visitors: Concerns/Pain Levels/Emotions:

Date: Caregivers:

Wake/Sleep

1	2	3	4	5	6	7	8	9	10	11	12	1	2	3	4	5	6	7	8	9	10	11	12

Toilet

Time:							
BM?							
Change?							

Meals: Water: ◊◊◊◊◊◊◊   Shower/Wash

Breakfast	AM snack	Lunch	PM snack	Dinner	Bedtime snack

Meds: ☐   ☐   ☐   ☐   ☐   ☐

Vitals:

Time	Blood pressure	Pulse	oxygen	Blood sugar		
	/					
	/					
	/					

Appointments or outings today: Future appointments or outings:

Visitors: Concerns/Pain Levels/Emotions:

Date: Caregivers:

Wake/Sleep

1	2	3	4	5	6	7	8	9	10	11	12	1	2	3	4	5	6	7	8	9	10	11	12

Toilet

Time:						
BM?						
Change?						

Meals: Water: ⬡⬡⬡⬡⬡⬡⬡   Shower/Wash

Breakfast	AM snack	Lunch	PM snack	Dinner	Bedtime snack

Meds: ☐   ☐   ☐   ☐   ☐   ☐

Vitals:

Time	Blood pressure	Pulse	oxygen	Blood sugar		
	/					
	/					
	/					

Appointments or outings today: Future appointments or outings:

Visitors: Concerns/Pain Levels/Emotions: